THE PROFESSIONAL GUINEA PIG

ROBERTO ABADIE

THE PROFESSIONAL GUINEA PIG

Big Pharma and the Risky World of Human Subjects

Duke University Press
Durham and London
2010

© 2010 Duke University Press

All rights reserved.

Printed in the United States of America on acid-free paper ∞

Designed by Heather Hensley

Typeset in Whitman by Keystone Typesetting, Inc.

Library of Congress Cataloging-in-Publication Data appear
on the last printed page of this book.

In loving memory of my mother Susana

CONTENTS

A NOTE ON METHOD

To protect informants I have chosen to identify them by pseudonyms. An exception is Robert Helms, who asked me to identify him by his real name. Anonymity is particularly important to avoid retaliation in cases when paid subjects are still active in clinical trials. The Community-Based Trial Organization (CBTO) is also a fictitious name. Despite my efforts, those knowledgeable about the AIDS institutional landscape in Philadelphia might be able to uncover the real site behind CBTO. I hope that nothing in this book compromises the mission of the organization. I could have gone further, concealing the identity of Philadelphia by referring to it only as a Northeastern city, but doing so would have deprived the reader of the full sociohistorical context in which this research is deeply embedded.

ACKNOWLEDGMENTS

It is a pleasure, as well as an obligation, to acknowledge all the individuals and institutions that made this book possible. First, to all those who opened their lives, shared memories, offered interpretations, and often challenged my own, enriching not only my work but more importantly, my life. Fortunately they are too many not to forget some, but my thanks to my roommate Michael from Fancy House, Robert Helms, Dave Onion, Frank Little, Jason, John, Spam, Scott, Shon, Mc Mike, Michael and Cidar Girl from Cidar House, Farmgirl at the Farm House, and James. Beyond the guinea pigs in West Philadelphia, I also want to thank the trust and commitment from King Lab Rat and the Canadian Guinea Pig.

At the Community-Based Trial Organization (CBTO) the director supported this project enthusiastically and made every effort to help me through it. The same can be said of all of its staff, its education coordinator, the nurses at the research department, and the members of the institutional review board. A special mention should be made of the CBTO's principal investigator, who encouraged me to pursue this research and who submitted graciously despite his tight schedule. Michael, Geraldine, John, and all the other patients deserve special thanks for their trust and disposition to share their very personal and sometimes painful recollections in a candid, open way, in order to help me get things right.

At the Graduate Center, City University of New York, Shirley Lindenbaum provided an inspirational model of scholarship, intellectual support, and kindness. Michael Blim, Ida Susser, and Don Robotham were dedicated mentors who contributed with their vivid interest and thoughtful critiques to bring to my attention key aspects of my work. I also owe a great deal of gratitude to former students and friends in the anthropology department. In particular Suzana Maia, Larissa Honey, Susan Falls, Erin Martineau, and Julian Brash engaged enthusiastically in discussing and providing valuable comments on numerous chapter drafts. Joseph Moses, David Vine, Nicole Laborde, and Lynn Horridge proved to be great colleagues and supportive friends.

At the Mayo Clinic I received enthusiastic support and encouragement from Barbara Koenig, Victor Montori, Molly Dingel, Marguerite Strobel, Jon Tilburt, Ashley Hicks, and Robbin Dawson.

Thanks to Betty Levin, Nicholas Freudneberg, and Barbara Weinstein at the Health Sciences Doctoral Programs, Graduate Center, for making me feel at home during my last phase of manuscript preparation.

Generous financial support gave me the time and ease to complete this project. Thanks to the Wenner-Gren Foundation for Anthropological Research for a four-year Wadsworth International Fellowship that made true my dream of becoming an anthropologist and supported me beyond coursework and into my fieldwork and writing. Pam Smith made me forget the more bureaucratic aspects of dealing with granting institutions, and I am very happy to be able to thank her for that. Thanks also to the Irving Horowitz Foundation for Social Policy that in 2005 provided support for my writing. Finally, a CUNY Writing Fellowship at Queens College during 2003–4 provided additional help.

At Duke University Press I had the enthusiastic guidance of my editor Miriam Angress and their dedicated staff and also benefited enormously from the comments and suggestions from Carl Elliott and Michael Oldani, the outside reviewers. This book is no doubt much better because of their combined efforts.

Writing this book has been an exciting intellectual journey, but it was not free of stress or anxieties. Luckily I was unconditionally supported by a close group of family and friends. Thanks to my extended Puerto Rican family in New York City: Tomas Noel, Monxo Lopez, Libertad Guerra, Camila Gelpi, Yesenia Aponte, Rebio Diaz, Ulla Berg, Macdara Valelly, and Vanessa Senati. From California my sister Cecilia, my two nieces Nicole and Angie, and my brother-in-law-Eduardo reminded me how much we love each other and what a long road we have traveled together. In Montevideo my sister Ximena, my nephew Santi, and my dad Roberto reminded me of what I left at home. From the other shore, in Buenos Aires, Daniel Zahra proved that it is possible to cultivate a friendship despite distance.

A GUINEA PIG'S WAGE

Risk, Body Commodification, and the Ethics
of Pharmaceutical Research in America

PROFESSIONAL RESEARCH SUBJECTS AND
THE NEW "ECONOMIES OF TORTURE"

On 16 June 2001 the national press first reported the death of Ellen Roche, a healthy twenty-four-year-old who had volunteered for an asthma study at Johns Hopkins University. The story revealed that a few days into the trial she felt very sick and was discharged and sent home. Within some hours she checked into the emergency room at a local hospital and fell into a coma. Ellen remained in this state until her death a month later. She had received $375 for participating in seven to nine sessions as an outpatient in a clinical drug study that resulted in her death (Altman 2001).

This tragic death—a dramatic one, but by no means unique—elicited responses from a variety of sources ranging from governmental agencies to self-proclaimed "bioethics experts." The federal government announced that it would interrupt all federal funding for biomedical research employing human subjects at Johns Hopkins until the university improved the protections for human subjects in research. In turn, Johns Hopkins agreed to review its informed-consent processes and addressed the claims of Ellen's relatives with out-of-court legal settlements. Commentators wrote about the event extensively in the press, focusing on whether institutional protections for human subjects volunteering in the trials were effective in protecting the volunteers' rights. Some inquired whether the volunteers understood the risks as they were framed in the informed-consent form. Others pointed to the increasing interrelationship between academic researchers and pharmaceutical companies. Their critiques were centered on conflicts of interest inside academic institutional review boards (IRBS) and the need to further regulate informed-consent processes to adequately safeguard volunteers' rights.

While critics made valuable remarks, one major point that they overlooked was that the volunteer was a healthy woman who had been paid to join a trial in which, apart from the monetary gain, there was no therapeutic benefit. Since the use of financial incentives to boost participants' enrollment is currently a significant trend in clinical trials research—in recent years the practice of offering some kind of financial compensation has been extended beyond phase I trials to later phases of drug development—I believe that there is a pressing need to address the consequences of increasing financial compensation for trial volunteers.

In fact, as this book will illustrate, being paid to test drug safety has become an essential part of the clinical drug trial enterprise in America. Pharmaceutical companies depend upon paid subjects to test an ever increasing number of drugs coming out of their "pipelines," and subjects see their participation not as an altruistic gesture but as their job, a particular kind of trade with some resemblance to a mild torture economy in which bodily pain, boredom, and compliance are exchanged for money (see the discussion of body commodification below). Spam, a resident of West Philadelphia in his early thirties and an experienced "guinea pig" who since quitting the trials has been working as a union organizer for janitors, offers his insight into what is it is like to participate in what he calls the torture economy as a paid subject:

> I don't know, another thing kind of funny too is that the manufacturing has been taken off, outside the country, so you are not allowed to do things any more. They call it the new economy, the informational economy. And the other side of this informational economy is the mild torture economy, you are not asked to produce or to do something anymore, you are being asked to endure something. So, if you are a guinea pig you are enduring something, people are doing things to you and you are just enduring it, you are not actually producing something. I feel that I am a worker but it is not work, it's like a security guard that does not produce nothing, just watches stuff. A security guard just gets paid to be bored, it's about how much can you deal with being bored,

that's the real hard part of it, the time and discomfort of being there. But it's different when you are in a cleaning job, I am doing something but being a guinea pig is just being paid to endure something that happens to me, which is weird. It's a different type of activity, I still feel that there is some work in it but the nature of work has changed. And I am letting people pay me in exchange for the control they have over me. (28 July 2004)

The participation of paid human volunteers in clinical trials research poses new problems that have not been analyzed thus far regarding financial compensation in trials research, risks, and the ethical regulations protecting human subjects. For example, does monetary compensation affect the way volunteers think about risks and benefits, placing volunteers at risk? Or might long-term participation in phase I trials increase risk awareness among professional guinea pigs? Are existing ethical frameworks enough to protect paid subjects, especially during the phase I trials? Finally, even if subjects are aware of the risks they face and even if their rights as subjects are ensured, are they not being exploited anyway as the weak link in the trial economy?

To answer these questions I conducted ethnographic research of paid research subjects in clinical trials conducted between July 2003 and December 2004 in Philadelphia. Its core was a group of self-defined professional guinea pigs who earned their livelihoods as research subjects testing the safety of drugs developed by the pharmaceutical industry. My work illuminates the professionalization of research subjects, the experiences and meanings associated with being a paid subject, the effects of financial compensation on the way volunteers understand and deal with risk, and the ethics of protecting human subjects in biomedical research. In addition, for comparative purposes I extended my research to a group of poor, mainly African American and Latino men and women testing HIV drugs and drug regimes for phases II and III at the Community-Based Trial Organization (CBTO).

New drug compounds are first tested in animals, usually dogs or rats—because the animals are cheap—and if the substance shows low toxicity it is then tested in phase I trials involving a small group of thirty to a hundred healthy human subjects. If the drug proves to be safe in phase I it then advances to phases II and III, which usually involve a much larger group of patients—sometimes in the thousands—who have the condition that the drug is supposed to improve. The compound continues to be tested for safety while its therapeutic value is assessed. Most compounds are abandoned during phase I because of their toxicity, and only a handful of drugs make it through all the research phases. The process of moving a drug from the lab to the public usually takes twelve to fifteen years. Making an accurate assessment of costs is more difficult, and the task has become deeply politicized amid efforts by the pharmaceutical industry to justify increasing drug prices: the industry routinely states that developing a new drug costs close to a billion dollars, whereas critics argue that costs are much lower and that significant amounts are spent not in research and development but on marketing exercises (see Angell 2004). In any case it is clear that after research and development are complete the costs of production are low, and that drugs that have made it into the market more than compensate the pharmaceutical industry for its research and development expenses, making it one of the most profitable industries in the country.

Payment to recruit healthy research subjects in America is a relatively new phenomenon. Until the mid-1970s phase I trials were conducted on prisoners, who in many ways were the ideal research subjects: captive, compliant, and readily available, with the prison setting providing an almost perfect controlled environment. But confinement, stigmatization, and financial need placed prisoners in a vulnerable position as research subjects (see chapter 6). Eventually abuses and renewed ethical concerns over the capacity of prisoners to give proper, uncoerced consent brought the practice to a halt.

The pharmaceutical industry was then forced to find a new population for an increasing number of drug trials. Paying healthy volunteers to test their drugs was the way to replenish the pool of research subjects. Initially students, artists, the unemployed, and other groups explored this new source of income. Some welcomed the opportunity and continued volunteering regularly. Not only did subjects become dependent upon the trial income but the drug companies increasingly appreciated having experienced trial subjects who were knowledgeable about the procedures and tolerated the depersonalization, pain, and boredom that so often accompany the trial experience. The pharmaceutical industry started luring these new subjects with even larger payments, mailings, and ads.

As a result, a new occupational category was developed: the professional guinea pig.

During my research I learned that in most cases the prospect of financial compensation is the guinea pigs' only motivation to participate in the trial economy. Drugs being tested range from compounds never tried before in men—"first-in-man" drugs, usually known to volunteers by a series of numbers and letters—to bioequivalence trials for drugs already on the market, like painkillers or psychiatric and other riskier drugs. According to Hogshire's estimates, in the early 1990s a volunteer could receive around $100 dollars a day as a research subject. Since then, financial compensation offered to volunteers in America has at least doubled (Hogshire 1992). In Philadelphia, a hotbed for clinical trials research, payment might range from $1,200 for three or four days in less intensive trials to $5,000 for three or four weeks in more extended ones; on occasion a trial might need even more time to be completed, with even higher payments going to volunteers. Trials that involve unusual and uncomfortable procedures or that test psychiatric drugs tend to pay more, in an attempt to attract reluctant research subjects.

Sometimes volunteers shift between their trial participation and low-paying jobs as cooks, construction workers, housepainters, or bike messengers. But for many participants trials become their full-time job: full-time volunteers might enroll in five to eight trials a year, deriving a total estimated income of $15,000 to $20,000 in exceptionally good years. Some experienced research subjects I met had participated in seventy, eighty, or even more phase I trials over the course of a few years. As one experienced professional guinea pig admitted, "You became addicted to the trials, to the easy money." This group, as this book illustrates, constitutes the backbone of phase I clinical trials in America and should be distinguished from other volunteers such as those affected by particular diseases or conditions, their kin, or even disease activists who volunteer only occasionally, motivated not by financial gain but altruistic, personal, or even political goals.

The trajectories of professional guinea pigs also contrast with those of HIV patients volunteering for later phases in clinical trials research. While for Michael, John, and Geraldine, poor patients enrolled in HIV trials at CBTO, "money helps"—although their participation does not command large sums of money like participation in phase I trials—but their motivation is not financial. As these histories illustrate, these volunteers hope to gain access to better heath care and expect the drug or regimes to offer them new therapeutic options while they learn more about their bodily responses to the virus. Their trial participation reveals itself as part of a larger strategy to control the disease that also involves an active role in managing their condition, "getting educated" about the virus, and having and open relationship with those who treat them. Volunteering in these trials is an additional resource in the fight for their lives, a powerful demonstration of the patients' will to live (Biehl 2007).

Paying healthy people to test for drugs that they don't need is another step toward commodifying the body in biomedicine. But unlike those who sell a kidney or plasma, professional guinea pigs see their whole bodies become the commodity. Trial subjects are well aware of how valuable their bodies are, despite the protestations of the pharmaceutical industry that subjects are volunteers being compensated just for their time. They see themselves as workers, entering a professional and contractual relationship with the industry. Trials are their business, a way of making quick, easy money.

Yet while dependent on the income, research subjects are generally distrustful of the pharmaceutical industry and resentful of the depersonalized, humiliating, and alienating treatment they often receive. Like workers in similar subaltern positions, professional guinea pigs both comply with the trial demands and resist them whenever they can, for example by introducing forbidden food or attempting to disrupt trial regimens. The industry counters these efforts by using financial inducements to recruit, retain, and control trial subjects. All volunteers in phase I trials whom I interviewed admitted that they had reservations about certain trials, such as those testing psychotropic drugs or drugs that alter sleep patterns or the immunological system—and for good reason—but they ended up volunteering anyway, swayed by the financial incentives. And once volunteers enter a trial, money is doled out strategically to ensure compliance: the largest sum is given after the trial is over, often with a bonus as an incentive for completion.

As my work illustrates, the prospect of financial gain shapes the way risk is understood and dealt with by professional guinea pigs. Paid subjects believe that most trials pose only a moderate risk. This perception is based on their personal experience as trial subjects and the rarity of serious adverse drug reactions (ADRs), but it is also influenced by their need to keep doing trials. I argue that social inequalities expose certain subjects to a disproportionate risk. Poor, disenfranchised volunteers face risks that they are unable or unwilling to recognize because of their need to earn a livelihood. This situation can be considered exploitative and directly challenges existing ethical regulations established to protect human subjects in biomedical research (Elliott 2008; Elliott and Abadie 2008). In a paradoxical turn, the prohibition against using prisoners in clinical trials created a new group of poor, vulnerable, and exploited population of healthy, paid subjects, this time a population created by the market. (As I will show in chapter 7, the creation of a professional class of paid healthy subjects recruited to test drug safety in phase I clinical trials challenges ethical arrangements established by the Helsinki Declaration of 1964 and the Belmont Report, issued in 1979 by the National Commission for the Protection of Human Subjects of Biomedical and Behavioral Research.) At the same time, neoliberal governance diminished the state's ability to protect the public and human subjects participating in clinical trials research by de-regulating the pharmaceutical industry. At least since the 1980s, the perceived need to create a "good business climate" has trumped previous regulatory concerns with consumers' and volunteers' well-being (Angell 2004).

The attempts of professional guinea pigs to manage risk are not completely successful. Many remain in trials for years, exposing themselves to potentially dangerous drug interactions and long-term effects. The organization of clinical trials and the lifestyle that guinea pigs lead make it difficult for them to become aware of these interactions and effects, which sometimes appear long after a trial is completed (Abadie 2009). In this respect guinea pigs differ from other workers in dangerous trades, such as coal miners and those exposed to asbestos or other industrial pollutants: although these workers were at first uninformed, after extended periods of sharing experiences they did become aware of the risks they faced, and of how these risks had been understated by the industry that employed them. (See Rosner and Markowitz 1988, which describes how silicosis emerged as an occupational disease in the early twentieth century after mining workers challenged industry and state-appointed experts.)

In the case of the professional guinea pigs, their mobility and relative anonymity conspire against this possibility. The fluidity and instability of the guinea pig workplace bring to mind the world of migrant agricultural workers, who face similar dangers caused by toxic substances. The lack of a centralized registry of human subjects who volunteer for phase I trials may also obscure the existence of problems for the pharmaceutical industry and regulatory agencies like the Food and Drug Administration (FDA). In addition, the pharmaceutical industry has no incentive to invest in research into long-term clinical-trials risks.

THE COMMODIFICATION OF THE BODY
IN CLINICAL-TRIALS DRUG RESEARCH

Recent technological advances in transplantation techniques, artificial reproduction, and drug development have resulted in the increasing commodification of the body (Scheper-Huges and Wacquant eds. 2002; Sharp 2000). Currently there is a local and international market for major organs like the heart, kidney, and liver, body tissue, reproductive material such as sperm and eggs, plasma, and even hair. As noted above, the whole body has also entered this market through the participation of paid research subjects in clinical-trials research. These are just a few examples of how bodies become commodified and integrated into a market economy.

In fact, as the anthropologist Leslie Sharp reminds us, this process of body commodification is not new in America, where corpses were long sold to dissectionists, anatomists, and surgeons. Other forms of commodification include the enslavement of human beings and the current use of reproductively rich products and tissues reaped from the dead (Sharp 2007, 42). One of the first to call attention to this issue was Karl Marx, who wrote, "A commodity appears at first sight an extremely obvious, trivial thing. But its analysis brings out that it is a very strange thing" (Marx 1976 [1867], 163). What Marx found strange is the obscuring of the exploitative labor processes that produced the commodity, making the commodity appear naturalized, with its own life independent from the social relations that originated it.

There has been recent scholarly interest in the commodification of the body in medicine (Sharp 2000; Scheper-Hughes 2000; Andrews and Nelkin 2001; Moore and Schmidt 1999). According to Sharp, organ transfer—like many new biotechnologies—elicits a powerful social anxiety among the public, which in turn leads to the industry's denial of body commodification. "Body commoditization—especially within the highly celebrated arena of organ transplantation—quickly erodes an already shaky public investment in medical trust. In response to such deep concerns, the transplant industry has generated an array of powerful euphemistic devices that obscure the commodification of cadaveric donors and its parts" (Sharp 2007, 17). Sharp notes that references to the commodification of the body are avoided by using the rhetorics of the "gift," through which organ transfers are equated with "donating life" and organs are "precious resources" to be "harvested." For Sharp these semantic choices make it possible to avoid referring to the trauma, suffering, and death involved in removing organs from donors. The language of the gift economy mystifies key aspects of organ transfer.

It is not only organ transplants that trouble American society. A similar anxiety can be detected in clinical-trials research. A popular novel by John Le Carré, *The Constant Gardener*, which describes the abuses of the pharmaceutical industry in conducting clinical trials among poor, disenfranchised African residents, raised numerous questions about the ethics of clinical trials in third world countries. The author criticized the pharmaceutical industry and also western governments and agencies for exploiting the poor for commercial and national gain and denounced the ethical abuses associated with clinical research in developing countries. While usually clinical trials in developed countries do not draw as much attention or provoke as much anxiety, concerns that the pharmaceutical industry might abuse volunteers in its search for profits were again brought to the fore by a recent "first-in-man" drug trial sponsored by Parexel in England in which six volunteers became seriously ill (Associated Press 2006).

As with organ transplantation, pharmaceutical corporations that conduct trials avoid referring to the commodification of the body in an attempt to maintain public trust. In clinical-trials research a discursive practice similar to the one observed by Sharp in connection with organ transfer contributes to the industry's denial of the commodification of volunteer's bodies. As we will see in chapter 2, the industry refers to trial subjects with the oxymoron "paid volunteer," the pretense being that they are compensated not for their labor but for their "time and travel expenses." Chapter 7 shows how language of informed consent obscures the risks of participation, for example by using euphemisms for death. Like the kin of organ donors, phase I volunteers resent and reject the industry's attempts to label them volunteers, insisting that they are professional guinea pigs.

"Commodities, like persons, have social lives," notes Arjun Appadurai (Appadurai 1986, 3). Marx understood this aspect of commodities, prompting us to consider what we might learn "if commodities could speak" (Marx 1976 [1867], 176). Professional guinea pigs, in opposition to most commodities and in particular to the drugs that they help to develop, do speak, and not just in a metaphorical sense. Volunteers' bodies become the site where the social and cultural processes that produced the emergence of professional subjects are articulated and displayed. As some authors have shown, embodiment adopts very particular forms (Csordas 1994; Lock and Farquhar eds. 2007). Many professional guinea pigs whom I met show some "battle scars." I was much impressed by KingLabRat's needle scars in both arms. Born to Puerto Rican parents and raised in Florida, he was a former soldier, drug dealer, and morgue worker in his late thirties who had been doing trials since his early twenties, touring the country in search of good trial opportunities. His pseudo-royal nickname mockingly referred to his years of trial participation. KingLabRat got his scars in the 1980s, a time when the use of catheters was discouraged to prevent the possibility of injury or infection, subjecting volunteers to innumerable needle punctures. Michael, my roommate, who started volunteering much later and had no needle marks in his arms, once showed me the scars on his back, product of a trial that required a biopsy. Pointing to them dismissively, he said: "I'll carry them forever. That's why [the pharmaceutical industry] pays so well." Although his scars were no bigger than an inch square, they reminded me of the cover of Allen Hornbum's book *Acres of Skin*, about experiments conducted on prisoners at Holmesburg Prison from the postwar era until the 1970s. In it a black man showed his back covered by large, decolorated skin patches, the product of a dermatological substance tested by a famous scientist from the University of Pennsylvania (Hornblum 1998).

But paid research subjects display more than their scars. As mindful bodies (Lock and Scheper-Hughes 1987), volunteers themselves offer accounts about what it means to be a professional guinea pig. One of the most important critiques of the pharmaceutical industry and the commodification of bodies in trials research is that the process not only exploits but dehumanizes research subjects. The tendency of research subjects to identify themselves with guinea pigs conveys well this notion of disembodied self. It is also not rare for volunteers to resort to images of torture, sex work, or prostitution when describing their activities. And their emergent solidarity as professionals—albeit professionals who perform a weird type of work, being paid to endure, as Spam notes—and their everyday forms of resistance at work draw attention to their efforts to reassert their human condition.

APPROACHING ANARCHIST GUINEA PIGS AND HIV VOLUNTEERS

I carried out eighteen months of ethnographic research in Philadelphia among research subjects volunteering in clinical drug trials. Philadelphia has historically been a major site for pharmaceutical research. The development of the pharmaceutical industry was shaped by its interaction with one of the earliest medical schools in the country (Silverman and Lee 1974), a process that provided a model for national and international developments in the field (Liebenau 1987). Large pharmaceutical companies such as GlaxoSmithKline (GSK), Wyeth, Bristol-Myers Squibb, and Merck began to operate and conduct research in the area. The city and its metropolitan area provide exceptional opportunities for enterprising professional subjects.

This ethnography focuses on a group of self-defined professional guinea pigs, all white males, who live in West Philadelphia in a community that could best be described as anarchist and volunteer mainly in the metropolitan area for phase I trials. Members of this community are articulate and vocal about their participation as trial subjects, the practices of the pharmaceutical industry, and the regulation of clinical trials, and their outspokenness helps to shape what Weinstein calls a public culture of guinea pigs (Weinstein 2001). They strongly object to the abuse and exploitation of clinical subjects in biomedical research but are also proud of the subjects' historical contribution to scientific progress.

One of the professional guinea pigs most experienced, articulate, and committed members, Robert Helms, had participated in more than eighty trials, mostly in the metropolitan area of Philadelphia, before being forced to stop a few years ago because of an imposed age limit of forty-five. A graduate in classical studies from Temple University and a former labor organizer in the health care sector, he edited *Guinea Pig Zero*, a zine dedicated to the experiences of professional human subjects, from 1996 to 2002. Its success led him to publish an anthology in 2002. Helms saw the publication, on which numerous local fellow guinea pigs collaborated, as an anarchist project intended to give voice to the experiences and concerns of professional human subjects in clinical-trials research. I was interested in the relationship between the clinical-trials experiences of this group of subjects and their views on social identity, risk, and body commodification. Just a few months before I met Helms, in the early days of my fieldwork, he and two other radical guinea pigs had played a key role in the first known strike at a phase I clinical trial at Jefferson Hospital, a research site that does clinical trials for the Merck pharmaceutical company. Helms was excited about this event when I first met him and asked me about it. The strike had been discussed in one number of GPZ and I was somewhat familiar with it. I realized that the strike and the role that the anarchist volunteers played in it opened an opportunity to explore not only issues related to their experiences of the trial but also their responses to some of the conditions they faced. This event reaffirmed my choice to study this group of volunteers, who became the main focus of my research.

It should be clear that this sampling of volunteers doing clinical trials research is not intended to be representative of the universe of those who participate in phase I research. The FDA publishes a list of all the drugs that received approval in a given year, but the pharmaceutical companies do not disclose the number of trials being performed or the number of volunteers enrolled. There is also no reliable information on the demographics of this population, and, as I have already mentioned, no centralized register of trial participants. Subjects remain essentially invisible, hidden.

While there are no demographic statistics about research subjects in phase I trials, most volunteers regularly enrolled in trials in the metropolitan area of Philadelphia are poor, relatively uneducated, and African American or Latino. In some trials white anarchists are a marginal presence, while in other trials they are not present at all. This overrepresentation of African Americans happens despite their historical misgivings about biomedical research and negative experiences dating back to the Tuskegee experiment (Jones 1981; Reverby ed. 2000). Anxieties among African Americans about participating in clinical research continue until the present, for example in connection with AIDS research (Jones 1981; Reverby ed. 2000; Epstein 1996).

While all professional volunteers share experiences and interests, racial and ethnic differences shape the way they understand and deal with risk, a topic that I wished to explore. I knew that many professional subjects travel across the country looking for trial opportunities, and while they do so they often stay at cheap hostels. I stayed at the youth hostel on Baker Street in downtown Philadelphia for my first month of fieldwork. There I met KingLabRat, with whom I lived at the hostel while witnessing his preparations for the trial. I sought any chance to interview him at key instances, from his initial trial screening to his discharge once the trial was over. We kept in touch, and I was able to join him months later when he came back to the city to enroll in a new trial. This case study offers a window into how race and ethnicity shape the experiences of professional guinea pigs outside the anarchist community of West Philadelphia. At the same time, I was aware that while males provide the standard of phase I clinical trials research, women have some occasions to participate as well. I also contacted women in this community, to assess if gender made any difference in the way they experienced their trial engagements.

Despite my focus on paid phase I subjects, I also studied HIV patients who volunteered in later phases of trial research to assess the safety and efficacy of pharmaceuticals or novel HIV drug regimes at CBTO. Since financial compensation has increasingly been extended to participants in the later phases of drug development, for comparative purposes I also extended the study to a group of HIV patients volunteering for phases II and III. Comparison between these participants and the phase I group illustrates the extent of body commodification in trials research and the particular problems of professionalizing the first phase of drug development. There are many important differences between these two groups of volunteers, the main one being that the phase I volunteers were healthy while volunteers for phases II and III had chronic and often life-threatening diseases. Members of both groups received some financial compensation for taking part in clinical trials. Professional guinea pigs in phase I trials might receive $200 to $400 for a day spent in a trial. Since most volunteers do two or three trials a year and some do six or more, their income can reach thousands of dollars. In contrast, HIV patients usually volunteer for one clinical trial and receive between $25 and $50 for a monthly visit in a trial that can last many years.

I contacted these patients as they came to the Research Division at CBTO for checkups, to have blood drawn, or to pick up trial medication. I had obtained approval from their local institutional review board for my research, which gave me a certain legitimacy. My informed consent forms had the institutional CBTO stamp, I used an office located inside the Research Division, and I was introduced by CBTO staff to incoming volunteers as a researcher doing a survey among patients volunteering at the facility. I have no doubt that while this institutional support helped me recruit many trial volunteers, modest financial compensation was also an incentive for many of those volunteers who contributed to my research.

I used various methods to collect and analyze data. I gathered data through a combination of participant observation and formal and informal interviews. My analysis relies on all sorts of data. In typical ethnographic fashion, eliciting my informants' comments on events and observing volunteers as they moved in and out of the trials and into their everyday lives was a central aspect of my research. I was precluded from volunteering as a subject myself by concerns for my well-being—strongly expressed by Shirley Lindenbaum, then my advisor, and many other faculty members—and by legal and regulatory constraints, which also prevented me from observing the routines, interactions, and activities of the clinical trials. In retrospect, choosing not to volunteer in trials as part as my data collection strategy proved to be the right decision, because I was able to retain some analytical and emotional distance while also being stimulated to think about additional sources of data with which to answer my research questions. So rather than firsthand knowledge, I relied on my observation of the professional guinea pigs' activities outside the trial locations. I was able to live with a group of them for more than a year in a very tight-knit community of professional research subjects and had ample opportunities to document in a lively and direct way their preparations for the trials, as well as their expectations, anxieties, and views. I followed prospective healthy subjects to their screening appointments, interviewed them after they had completed the first portion of the trial—usually after a week or so, usually as inpatients—and again at the end of the trial. The goals, risks, and benefits of a trial are typically disclosed to participants mainly in the consent form that they sign after enrollment. Discussing the information contained in these documents in a naturalistic setting, soon after the volunteers had signed them, afforded a unique window into their perspectives on risk and how it relates to financial compensation.

In addition to participant observation, I conducted more than forty semi-structured interviews, approximately half with self-defined professional guinea pigs volunteering in phase I trials and half with HIV patients in the community site. This technique allowed me to explore the topics of financial compensation, risk perception, and risk management. While this method was useful for capturing general views about the ways risks are perceived and dealt with by subjects, it cannot account for individuals' experiences of the trials and how they change over time. For this I conducted twelve life stories, having chosen from among the participants according to the following criteria: length and frequency of participation, types of trials in which the participant had volunteered, and risks experienced during previous trials, if any. I inquired about the participants' personal experiences in clinical trials and their understanding of risks, focusing on the relationship between the participants' experiences of trials, their possible changes in risk awareness and risk management, and their expectation of financial gain.

My fieldwork was facilitated by my experience as a guinea pig. Although I did not take part in clinical trials during my research in Philadelphia, during the last months of 1998, while I was pursuing my MA in anthropology at the Université Laval in Quebec City, I volunteered on a couple of occasions for a major contract research organization (CRO) that conducted phase I trials for several local and international pharmaceutical companies which had their headquarters a few blocks away from my campus. At that time I never imagined that this could be a topic of academic interest and I volunteered only for the money. I found out about the trials from radio and newspaper ads that invited healthy young males with free time to make "quick, easy money" by becoming paid volunteers for clinical drug research. Since kindergarten I had always been wary of needles, and the idea of selling my body to the pharmaceutical industry gave me pause. However, unable to work in a foreign country and in need of cash, I ended up accepting the invitation.

The research facility was a functional, flat, uninviting five-story building, no doubt a fine expression of the Soviet architecture of the 1960s and 1970s that also shaped the university campus. The research floor was crowded; dozens of double bunk beds were aligned in facing rows. A yellow light went on at night after the regular lights went off. I couldn't avoid noticing the resemblance to a prison cell. For a minute I was reminded of abuses involving prisoners and other vulnerable populations used as research subjects in the past. However, I decided not to focus on the risks involved in becoming a trial subject and thought instead of the money I would get. The ad line "quick, easy money" still resonated in my mind.

Most paid subjects whom I met were frequent trial participants who defined themselves as "professionals." Volunteers were a mix of mentally disabled persons trying to supplement their governmental disability checks, university students after tuition money, artists buying some creative time, and generally unemployed or unemployable subjects who would waste no time putting the cash to good use. In a way that resembled the mob practices depicted in *The Sopranos* more than the careful accounting of a research institution, cash was handed to us on the last day, at discharge, in yellow envelopes. (More than a decade later, the conditions at clinical trials sites in Canada seemed not to have changed that much. See Martin Patriquin 2009.)

The first drug I tested was a new version of a drug already on the market that combats heartburn and gastritis. I learned later that the drugs tested in these trials are called "me too drugs" and are preferred by paid subjects because the drug has already been tested in research and used by patients, providing additional security. For a five-day inpatient study I received $550 Canadian. The second trial was a new drug to increase appetite in terminal patients with HIV or cancer. This experimental drug was a "first-in-man" because it was the first time the compound was tested in human beings, having been tested for safety in dogs and rats. It did not increase my appetite, but the trial definitely contributed to augmenting my diminished bank account by $800. I am sure in retrospect that the "financial compensation for my time and travel" did not fully compensate for the risks I faced, the pain of endless blood extractions, and the boredom of spending hours doing nothing but watching TV.

Having volunteered as a paid human subject for a couple of phase I clinical trials, I had a particular insight into the lives of volunteers. Our shared experiences and sensibilities allowed other volunteers to interact with me at a common level of understanding and trust. I had a point of entry into their views and feelings not accessible by other research methods, such as questionnaires and semi-structured interviews.

While my ethnography focuses on paid human volunteers in clinical-trials research, I also intended to grasp the scientist's understanding of and dealings with risks and ethics in a context of increasing commoditization. CBTO provided a good starting point. Its principal investigator is in charge of all trials sponsored by the pharmaceutical industry and was extremely supportive of my research from the beginning. I conducted extensive interviews with him to explore risk perception, risk management, and commodification in clinical trials used to develop new drugs and drug regimes for HIV patients. In addition, since I had to obtain approval for my research from CBTO's institutional review board, I was invited to make my case to the board and interviewed the IRB's chair and other members to discuss how they saw issues of risks, the protection of human subjects, and commodification in relation to the research being conducted at this community-based trial site.

ANTHROPOLOGICAL CONTRIBUTIONS

The emergence of professional research subjects who volunteer to test experimental drugs are an example of what Michaela di Leonardo terms the "exotic at home." Professional guinea pigs are an exotic development of technological and medical culture, with their own ethos, identities, and practices. This book is an attempt to further consider di Leonardo's call for an anthropological examination of phenomena that are "hidden in plain sight around us" (di Leonardo 1998, 10). My research calls attention to hidden problems brought about by the increasing commodification of the body in clinical trials, in the context of an emerging professional subjectivity created by new regimes of techno-science and capital accumulation (Rajan 2005; Rajan 2006; Rose 1996; Rose 2006). Thus far this topic has failed to capture the imagination of anthropologists. My research is the first ethnographic description of the experiences of healthy paid subjects in the United States, or anywhere.

Even so, pharmaceuticals in general have not escaped the notice of anthropologists, who have explored the commodity chain from production sites to the uses of pharmaceuticals by consumers (Petryna, Lakoff, and Kleinman 2006). They have also looked at marketing practices, the role of drug representatives in shaping doctors' prescription practices (Oldani 2004), and the cultural, economic, and political determinants of drug consumption (Abraham 1994; Biehl 2007; Farmer 2002). And although anthropologists have paid little attention to the first phase of clinical drug trials (Whyte, vand der Geest, and Hardon 1996; Whyte, vand der Geest, and Hardon 2002), they have studied the pharmaceutical industry's increasing reliance on CROs to run the daily operations of trial sites, including the recruitment of volunteers and the hiring of friendly IRBs to speed up drug development in the United States (Fisher 2009) and abroad, mainly in third world countries, where regulations are few or unenforced (Petryna 2006; Petryna 2009). Documenting the professionalization of clinical-trials subjects in the first phase of drug development represents a contribution to the emergent field of the anthropology of pharmaceuticals.

This book is based on classic ethnographic research, documenting the discourses and practices in the particular historical and sociocultural context in which research subjects live and make decisions about trials, money, risks, and benefits. Its situated knowledge is one of the strengths of anthropological inquiry, offering a description of the forces leading to the professionalization of trial subjects in phase I clinical research as well as the meanings, emotions, and everyday struggles involved in guinea-pigging. By exploring the sociocultural processes that transform bodies into valuable commodities as research subjects, this ethnography directly contributes to the anthropological study of the body (Lock 1992; Lock and Scheper-Hughes 1987; Lock and Farquhar eds. 2007; Martin 1994) and body commodification (Sharp 2000; Sharp 2007; Scheper-Hughes 1996; Scheper-Hughes and Wacquant eds. 2004). It also furthers the literature on risk by emphasizing how commodification processes shape professional subjects' understandings and responses to risk. The richness of ethnographic data also illuminates current debates on biocitizenship (Petryna 2002; Rose 2006) and the ethics of protecting human subjects in clinical trials and more broadly in biomedical research. My aim is to advance ethical discussions which are often presented in a largely formal, individualistic, rational, and legalistic framework, and it seeks to contribute to an approach that incorporates the cultural context in which individuals make decisions about risks and benefits (Levin 1985; Marshall 1992; Marshall and Koenig 2004).

Finally, while conducting normative analysis and formulating policy recommendations are not the main foci of my work, I engage in some of each here in the hope of stimulating public debate, with the goal of transforming public policies to ensure the ethical and safe engagement of paid subjects in trials research.

The reader will come to understand the experiences of a group of self-defined professional guinea pigs who earn their livelihoods as research subjects for phase I clinical trials by testing drugs being developed by the pharmaceutical industry. By following research subjects as they volunteer, the book illustrates the social organization of clinical trials, the role of financial compensation, and its effects on the ethical arrangements intended to protect human subjects in biomedical research.

The Introduction presents the aim of my research, the research problem and question, and relevant theoretical and methodological data. Chapter 1 explores the social organization of clinical-trials drug research and describes how increasingly large payments to subjects reinforce professionalization among trial volunteers. Chapter 2 deals with the identity, ideology, compliance, and resistance of trial subjects. Chapter 3 illustrates the way paid subjects understand and deal with the risks involved in being a professional guinea pig. Chapter 4 provides a counterpoint to previous chapters by describing the social organization of phase II and III trials for HIV pharmaceuticals at a community-based research organization. Chapter 5 portrays the life stories of Michael, John, and Geraldine, illustrating the struggles and aspirations of poor HIV patients enrolled in trials at a community-based research organization. Chapter 6 describes the history of the development of pharmaceutical clinical trials in America. Chapter 7 revisits the central questions about paying subjects to volunteer in clinical-trials research. Chapter 8 summarizes research findings and offers public policy recommendations to improve the safeguards afforded to professional guinea pigs.

1

GUINEA-PIGGING

The In/Formal Economy of Phase I Clinical Trials in Philadelphia

EXPERIMENTATION

Phase I clinical trials employ healthy human volunteers to test new drugs under development by the pharmaceutical industry, not for therapeutic efficacy but for drug safety. Phase I trials are designed to assess the safety of the drug or compounds being tested, and represent the first time a chemical compound is tested in human beings after having been tested in laboratories and then in animals. After a drug proves its safety in phase I it goes through phases II and III, which involve larger groups of volunteers. While phase II also continues to test the drug for safety, this phase and the next one are intended to test for therapeutic benefits. If the drug proves safe and therapeutically efficacious, it then receives FDA approval and goes on the market.

Phase I clinical trials are designed as controlled experiments that follow an experimental design. The trials are devised to obtain information about how the human body responds to a particular substance, what the levels of toxicity are, and how the drug is absorbed and eliminated. As previously mentioned, this phase is not designed to test therapeutic effects on the volunteers. It is for this reason that the trials have also been described as "non-therapeutic" in contrast to the "therapeutic" trials in phases II and III.

RECRUITMENT, RETENTION, AND PROFESSIONALIZATION OF HUMAN SUBJECTS

Clinical-trial researchers need to recruit volunteers to carry out trials. A healthy population is an indispensable requirement of the experimental design employed in randomized clinical trials (RCTs) used in phase I clinical-trials research.

A healthy and homogeneous trial population would ensure that all participants have the same condition at the outset, making it easy to attribute the outcome of the experiment to the drug regimes to which the volunteers are exposed. Therefore, the lack of any existing medical condition is an indispensable requirement for the realization of any clinical trial. Phone interviews screen medical histories, as do further screenings to select the candidates and again at the beginning of the trial. A healthy population also contributes to minimize risks among volunteers by eliminating potential drug interactions with existing medical conditions.

Pharmaceutical researchers not only need to recruit a sufficient number of healthy volunteers to conduct trials but need to do so quickly. The more time they expend in finding the volunteers they need, the more they delay their scheduled experiments. Delays are costly and add to overall research expenditures. Obtaining the right number of volunteers but with the wrong qualifications also puts the trial's outcome at risk, seriously compromising the volunteers' health and the validity of the trial. But recruiting the right number and the right kind of volunteers is no easy task. That is why in recent years there has been a shift in the way phase I trials are conducted. While some pharmaceutical companies still run their own trials, most have been outsourced to universities, or to independent contractors known as CROs.

During phase I the professional knowledge required in drug development is mostly supplied by biostatisticians and experts in toxicology. In contrast to later phases in drug research, no specialized knowledge about a particular disease or medical condition is required, making the task of outsourcing easier. Speed, flexibility, and the ability to recruit a large number of volunteers are the usual presentation cards for aspiring CROs. Their functions are broad, from recruiting volunteers and gathering data to ensuring ethical oversight of the trials with the help of a usually friendly ad hoc IRB.

In an open, competitive market, CROs compete among themselves, trying to lure the best research subjects they can find. In recent years increasing competition to attract subjects in high-demand areas has led to a surge in the amounts paid to volunteers. But financial inducements are only part of the package offered to prospective subjects. Instead of the prisonlike environment offered ten or more years ago, now there are individual suites, Internet access, flat-screen televisions, and even pool tables, among other amenities. Food has also improved, along with a more professional and "respectful" staff. Because of their anti-consumerist tendencies anarchist guinea pigs are not generally appreciative of fancy sites, which usually involve a large number of trial subjects and rotating personnel. Many told me that these sites look like factories, large and impersonal, furthering their sense of alienation. They prefer trials at Jefferson, an academic hospital with a very friendly and stable staff but less glamorous facilities, and some guinea pigs, like Helms, had volunteered only there in recent years. KingLabRat and the Canadian Guinea Pig, in contrast, found large sites like those of GSK very nice and volunteered there quite often. Of course investments in amenities are only made where they are really necessary to attract or retain paid subjects. In remote areas, such as parts of the Midwest, where demand for volunteers is not as strong and paid subjects have fewer choices, trial conditions are not as good.

A glimpse at just a few of the hundreds of advertisements published in weekly newspapers in Philadelphia, or posted at recruitment sites at the major pharmaceutical companies operating in the area, summarizes industry requirements for phase I clinical trials. Subjects must be healthy males eighteen to forty-five years old with flexible schedules. The companies offer "financial compensation for time and travel expenses" or, more directly, invite the volunteer to "make money" by joining a trial. It is not hard to see the gender bias in pharmaceutical research. In phase I clinical trials males have historically been the preferred human subjects and remain so. The gender bias in recruiting volunteers is not lost among paid female volunteers: "When I started doing trials they were not for women at all and I remember that a doctor told me that recently had been a study at that place for a breast cancer medication and the volunteers were all men. I asked why and she said it was because the pharmaceutical industry still thinks of men as normal humans and women as aberrations. Women have abnormal bodies because they are not men, men are the norm. Now most of the trials if you are sterile women can do them, so I think that this is their main concern with it" (Cidar House Girl, 12 June 2004).

Since the level at which an experimental drug becomes toxic is unknown—that is precisely what a study is to determine—the pharmaceutical industry fears that experimental drugs might affect fertility and pregnancy outcomes in women who volunteer for phase I trials, exposing the industry to lawsuits. Despite this, the pharmaceutical industry has been encouraged in the last decade to incorporate a more diverse population in trials. Still, while women have been included in phase I trials research, they are a very marginal population. Most of the trials enroll only men and just a few recruit both men and women. Trials intended to assess the toxicity of contraceptive drugs or other products devised for women's use employ female volunteers, which is no doubt an advance if we consider—for example—that the birth control pill was originally tested in men.

DEMAND FOR HEALTHY BODIES

Toxicological trials are not seeking just any men but "healthy" men. Again, the recruitment ads give us some clues: "not smoker," "drug-free," "non-congenital conditions," "takes no medication." The pharmaceutical industry goes to great lengths to make sure that the volunteers recruited for phase I trials are "healthy" and thus appropriate research subjects. Phase I trials depend not only on recruitment but also on retention. If someone withdraws from a trial before it is complete for whatever reason, the validity of the trial may be compromised. In sum, market recruitment ensures the availability of the large number of subjects the industry needs to perform phase I clinical trials while also contributing to the correct operation of the trial.

Professional volunteers are aware of the key role that they play in ensuring that clinical trials are run smoothly:

> Well, the biggest thing with a clinical trial is that it's a poker game. The clinical trial wants a specific person with a specific profile that doesn't exist. They know it; guinea pigs know it and people don't talk about it. They want a person that is very healthy, has an open schedule, under a certain weight but does not exercise. A lot of times they ask you not to exercise because that messes up with the trial but then they want you to be under certain weight. The perfect volunteer they require doesn't exist. Everybody lies about complying and that's the biggest thing. I lied about my family medical history, yeah, about drug use, taking medicine. They have a lot of pressure to recruit enough people. The

recruiters are under a lot of pressure to recruit, they need people. And also, once they found you too, they want you to continue. Once you showed dependable, you did the study and went through the whole thing, when they need to do a blood draw your veins work, you pee when they tell you to pee, never complain, once they have that they want to keep you. (Spam, 28 July 2004)

Paid volunteers are well aware of the demand for an idealized, perfectly healthy volunteer. They also realize that their body is a valued commodity in clinical trials research. Certainly, as Spam observes, it is not an abstract body that is sought and rewarded in phase I trials, but a well-trained, disciplined, and complying body—or subject.

There is no clear guinea pig career. Some volunteers started their career by selling blood or modeling for art schools, or doing less invasive procedures such as MRIS. Others jumped right into trials. Most guinea pigs have done exclusively trials or moved quickly into trials. This trajectory seems to support the idea that blood, semen, and other body fluids are not as valuable as body as a whole.

Financial compensation plays a central role in recruiting and retaining volunteers. The payment is scheduled to maximize the chances of ensuring compliance with the research protocol among volunteers. Generally it takes at least two or three weeks from the first phone interview to the time a trial begins. It is not until the first leg of the trial is over, or the whole trial if it is a short one, that the volunteer gets paid. Volunteers leaving the trial before the first leg of the trial is completed do not receive any payment, unless they can prove that they are experiencing serious adverse affects as a consequence of their participation. Since the object of the trial is to study the toxicity of the drug, side effects are expected, and therefore volunteers may have a difficult time negotiating their paid discharge with the trial staff. If the volunteers are successful in making their point, then they get paid based on the number of days they stayed in the trial.

There are a number of ways the industry promotes professionalization among human subjects volunteering for their clinical trials. All major research sites in metropolitan Philadelphia have a database of previous volunteers from which they draw when they need to fill a new trial. Potential volunteers regularly receive announcements of forthcoming trials. Registered volunteers can also check the industry's web site for trial opportunities. Some, like Michael, make occasional phone calls to inquire about possible trials and to let recruiters know about their availability. Most research sites offer financial incentives for referrals, usually from $50 to $100. After a new volunteer finishes a trial successfully the volunteer who referred him gets a check. Eager to fill slots, research sites attempt to recruit volunteers for forthcoming trials even before a clinical trial is over. Currently volunteers are required to wait one month after they have finished a trial before submitting to screening in a new trial, but participants usually receive "invitations" for screenings in future trials once the waiting period is over. This waiting period is intended to "wash out," or eliminate, any trace of a drug from an earlier study. Yet only a few days after a drug has been taken it usually cannot be detected in a blood test. Some people who participated in trials in the early 1980s—when regulations imposing a waiting period between trials were almost nonexistent—remember that even before finishing one trial volunteers were invited to screen for a forthcoming trial and if accepted were enrolled right away.

A PROFESSIONAL GUINEA PIG TRIAL'S JOURNEY

"I needed money and some friends that do trials told me about this one coming. My friend told me that I should sign up because it paid really well for not having to do a lot. It turned out that the drugs weren't too risky and so for the money that you were making it was a pretty safe bet." That's how Michael, my roommate at Fancy House, described how he entered his last trial, just a couple of days after I moved there in early February 2004. He was a twenty-five-year-old white Kansan who had moved to Philadelphia and to Fancy House, one of dozens of radical, anarchist communes in the West section of the city at that time.

Although Michael had a degree in art design and did occasional under-the-table commissions designing jewelry and clothing for some friends in New York, this was not his main source of income. He had been a bike messenger first and later worked in the kitchen of a catering firm. When I met him he had just cut one side of his right thumb while operating a slicing machine. The cut was deep and painful, the kind of wound that made it impossible to stitch. Having no health insurance, Michael dealt with it by washing the site with disinfectants and removing the bandages from time to time. He missed a couple of days at work and then went back to his catering job, but not for long. He had earlier volunteered for a clinical trial, and two weeks before his accident with the slicing machine he had called one of the oldest medical schools in the city to find out if there were any clinical trials for which he could volunteer. He called not once but twice. As he told me: "You have to keep calling until they know who you are. They have a lot of people interested. I gave them the names of two people that I knew who were regular trial participants there. That helped me out."

The trial comprised two six-day periods with a washout period of ten days in between. For the duration of the trial Michael would need to comply with some restrictions, including prohibitions against drinking grape juice or exercising heavily, because these activities interfere with the drug regime. Michael's trial is a typical double-blind placebo trial, or randomized clinical trial (RCT), in which participants are randomly assigned to different groups that are administered different drug regimes. He had been placed in one of six groups receiving a combination of placebo and different drug regimes varying from 0.4 mg to 10 mg, and he would not know which drug regime he would receive. To test the safety and efficacy of the drug, he would get a tetanus vaccine and then have a biopsy performed to assess the anti-inflammatory response. Michael would have a total of five biopsies during the trial.

After calling a couple of times and naming names Michael was granted a phone interview that lasted about thirty minutes and covered questions about his health history, diet, smoking habits, drinking, and illegal substance consumption habits. As noted above, any congenital disease, mental health problems, or admission of regular use of alcohol or illegal substances is enough to disqualify a potential candidate. In addition, a few extra pounds, low or high blood pressure, or a contaminated urine or blood sample is enough to exclude a prospective volunteer. Some research sites ban prospective volunteers for life if a "toxic" substance is found during the screening process, while others make the ban temporary.

With such requirements, recruiting enough volunteers for toxicological research is not an easy task for the pharmaceutical industry. Since clinical trials use a controlled diet that includes meat, self-identified vegetarians are also banned from clinical trials. Having done clinical trials before, Michael knew that he could not be honest about his vegetarian diet. He passed the phone screening and was then called to do an in-person screening for a trial a few days later. Prospective volunteers won't know which trial they will be participating in until they pass the screening process. Michael's screening lasted one hour and involved blood and urine tests, an electrocardiogram, and measurement of his height, weight, and body mass index. Michael had to sign an informed-consent form for the blood draws and other tests. The screening is very demanding, and any minor deviation from the requirements may exclude a volunteer. Luckily for Michael, a few days afterward he received a call from the recruiter informing him that he had passed the screening tests and was accepted.

The next day Michael went back to the hospital, where a nurse practitioner showed him the informed-consent form describing in detail what the study was about, how long it was going to last, the schedule, and financial compensation. He had the opportunity to ask questions about the trial, the drug being tested, and possible risks. He read the informed-consent carefully, asked questions, and then took the twenty-page document home and kept reading it. He wasn't supposed to sign it then but at the beginning of the trial a few days later.

After his screening session Michael received more information about the trial that he would volunteer for. It was an eleven-week, outpatient trial of a new anti-inflammatory drug for which he would receive $1,700. The study was designed to test the safety of the drug. The trial involved three groups of approximately eight volunteers each; a maximum of thirty volunteers would be recruited.

Five days after he qualified, Michael showed up at 7:30 in the morning at Jefferson to start the trial. After signing the informed-consent document he had a new round of checkup tests: "The same thing [as in the screening tests a few days ago], because they wanted to make sure that everything is current," Michael told me. He also had his first biopsy: staff removed skin from his back, with local anesthesia, and then two stitches closed the wound. At 2:00 in the morning he was awakened for additional tests, but was not given any drugs.

He "dosed," that is, took the drug, the following morning at 9:30. "It's just a couple of pills and then we swallow and they check if we swallow them, look into your mouth and into your tongue and everything." Every patient doses at the same time every day. After dosing Michael had his blood drawn. Staff members use a catheter to draw five or six vials. While Michael was at Jefferson, staff identified him by his tag number, 8246, although informally many nurses would address him by name. Of the seven people in his group Michael knew five. He spent his time at the lounge, watching TV, playing video games, watching movies, and just hanging around. He spent the first night at the hospital, then left the next evening to return the next morning. The days when he just dosed and had blood drawn he spent less time at the hospital than when he underwent biopsies. Six days into the trial he began the ten-day washout period, without any dosing or blood draws. Michael came back at the end of this period for the second part of the trial: another six days of dosing, blood draws, and occasional biopsies. After a few days he felt confident that he would finish the trial and receive the money, so he quit his catering job for good. He received a quarter of the financial compensation after the first phase was over and the remaining amount at the end. Michael didn't seem to worry about the scars left on his back by the biopsies: "I'll carry them for the rest of my life," he told me matter-of-factly.

After cashing his trial's check Michael spent the money on a new, state-of-the-art laptop computer. He was confident about getting into another trial as soon as the thirty-day waiting period between trials expired. He intends to do two more trials to save enough money to be able to live in Spain for a year without the need to have a full-time job there. Broke in the meantime, he distributed lists for a Democratic candidate during a couple of weekends in the neighborhood for $10 an hour and managed to hold on until his next trial with the income he received after a week of showing car models at a horse fair in Pennsylvania.

DEMOGRAPHICS OF THE PROFESSIONAL RESEARCH SUBJECTS

I surveyed eighteen people participating in at least one paid phase I clinical trial in Philadelphia. Their ages ranged from twenty-one to forty-six. Most of the volunteers were in their mid- to late twenties. All but four volunteers were men. Ethnically most volunteers self-identified as white or Caucasian; one volunteer self-identified as Latino.

The volunteers' educational levels covered a wide range: one did not finish high school, four finished high school, six did some undergraduate study, six finished an undergraduate degree, and one was enrolled in doctoral studies. Only three of the volunteers owned their own house, but in all three cases the owners shared the property communally. The large majority lived in communal houses but did not own them and paid rent. Most did not have any kind of health coverage. Just three had HMO coverage provided by their current employers.

When asked about their motives to enter the trial, volunteers without exception declared that trials were the opportunity to "make easy money," "quick money," "a considerable amount of money in a relatively short amount of time," "a huge sum."

"SOUNDS LIKE A VACATION!"

Survey findings confirm that financial incentives are very important in shaping volunteers' decisions to enroll in phase I clinical trials. Only two volunteers mentioned an altruistic motive along with the financial incentives, and these were volunteers who were not part of the "guinea pigs" community based in West Philly: their social backgrounds were different, and they also differed in their views of the ethics and politics of clinical-trials research.

Financial gain is also reflected in the volunteers' response to a survey question about their main motivation for taking part in the trial. As noted, all the volunteers pointed to financial benefit as their main consideration, but they also noted the duration of the studies and their location. The risk level was mentioned by some as a disincentive, and if a trial was perceived as risky, volunteers said that they would not participate regardless of the financial incentives. I discuss risk perception in depth in chapter 3.

Frank Little, a young volunteer who had done just a couple of trials, sums it up well:

> I was working as a carriage driver for a while downtown and it was OK money but then I saw the paychecks that my friends were doing with the clinical studies. Floyd and Jason told me that they did lots of money. It varies from study to study but it was a significant amount of money for not very much time and what these guys actually had to do for the study is to lie in bed, get one or two pills, watch TV, read, play board games, and periodically have their blood drawn. Periodically they also had to give urine samples and they get this huge chunk of money. I said: "except for the needles and the pills it sounds like a

vacation!" The blood draws vary from study to study but, you know, they said frequent blood draws but I didn't care about that, for the amount of money that we are getting in compensation getting my blood drawn a few times is something that I can sacrifice. It's much better than working eight, twelve hours a day just to get my blood drawn five, six times a day [laughs]. (Frank Little, 9 December 2004)

Since money plays such an important role in the volunteers' experience it is not surprising that volunteers should be so candid when they talk about it. Money is one of their main topics of conversation when they talk about trials. Volunteers are always interested in finding new trial opportunities. Usually the conversation focuses on the best forthcoming trials in the area and the financial compensation offered.

When paid volunteers refer to a trial they have completed or one that they might want to join, they always identify the trial by the amount of money offered. Sometimes they also note the duration, whether the trial is inpatient or outpatient, and the drug being tested. Descriptions by sponsors offer information about the physical location of trials. They would say something like this: "A $3,000, two-week, inpatient [or outpatient] trial for a first-in-man drug with such-and-such sponsor." Volunteers are aware of the financial potential of each trial and are able to compare daily and even hourly earnings. Volunteers use these ratios to make decisions among competing trials. All things being equal, the trials that pay more per day or hour are preferred. As a rule, *Guinea Pig Zero*, the zine for professional human subjects edited by Helms and reflecting the views of anarchist volunteers in Philadelphia, advises potential volunteers to turn down any inpatient trial that pays less than $200 a day in the Philadelphia metropolitan area.

Clinical trials for phase I drugs in metropolitan Philadelphia typically offer between $200 and $400 a day to volunteers. Compensation for engagement in a trial might range between $1,200 for three or four days in less intensive trials to $5,000 for three or four weeks in more extended ones; exceptionally a trial might need even more time to be completed.

Volunteers are not compensated for the time they spend in the phone interview, but most of the research sites offer a small amount, $25 or $30, to volunteers for their participation in the screening. Volunteers often receive a voucher for a meal at the hospital cafeteria after the screening and when they make their occasional follow-up visits to the research site. Volunteers are also compensated for being alternates. Alternates spend the first night of a trial on-site in case any volunteer in the trial cannot continue to participate. Usually the alternate walks away the next morning, having been paid $100 without having taken any drug or undergone any blood draws or intrusive procedures. Alternates are then scheduled to participate in the next cohort of the trial, thus gaining an additional payment.

BETTER THAN A JOB AT MCDONALD'S

Participation in inpatient clinical trials is time-intensive, demanding the volunteer's presence in a particular location for the duration of the trial. Mixed trial regimes that balance inpatient with outpatient visits are less demanding but still limit the volunteer's use of free time during the trial. Volunteers are required to have a flexible job schedule or not work at all at the time of enrollment. As many volunteers admitted, the independence and flexibility, not to mention the income, afforded by participating in clinical trials was much better than a job at McDonald's.

The requirement for a flexible schedule is reflected in the occupational status of the volunteers interviewed. Eleven of the eighteen said that they had worked, in addition to participation in clinical trials research, and seven had trials as their only source of income at the time they were interviewed. Among those who declared they were employed, only three held full-time jobs, while the other eight worked part-time. Of those who held full-time jobs two were labor organizers (one working to organize supermarket workers; the other, janitors) and one held two jobs (repairing bikes at a cooperative bicycle store and selling books at a children's bookstore).

The jobs of the volunteers who worked part-time were diverse. Most were independent, blue-collar jobs such as construction worker, painter, bike messenger, house or office cleaner, housekeeper, and cook. Three volunteers worked part-time at the Wooden Shoe, the oldest anarchist bookstore in the city, which is run as a co-op. The large majority in the sample self-identified as "blue collar" or "working class." Some had working-class parents; others chose typical working-class occupations. No doubt their anarchist ideology, with its emphasis on independent, non-exploitative labor, played a role in their choice of occupation as well as in their class identification.

Professional guinea pigs realize the difficulties they face in depending exclusively on clinical trials for income. While living in the Philadelphia metropolitan area affords a regular supply of opportunities for participation in clinical trials research, the demands of the RCT make eventual enrollment unpredictable and unreliable. Urine and blood samples can be contaminated, not just by illegal substances but by bacteria found in the testing lab. Even if the samples are not contaminated, their values can be too high or too low, thus preventing the candidate from entering the trial. Sometimes a small variation in diet or exercise produces certain enzymes that show up in the samples, disqualifying the candidate. Even high or very low blood pressure can prevent candidates from entering a trial. Certainly there are many other contingencies that conspire against the enrollment of a perspective volunteer and are beyond the volunteer's ability to control. Anticipating rejection, volunteers often screen for two trials simultaneously. Despite their efforts to gain entry, the stringent screening process often bars volunteers for months at a time. Being a full-time guinea pig demands a great deal of energy from volunteers. Scott, an experienced guinea pig, describes his first years working exclusively as a research subject and his later shift between trials and formal employment:

> I just moved to Philadelphia about ten years ago now and I didn't want to go back to a regular job. I traveled that summer, went back to Minnesota and came back here and was looking for a way of making money that was easy and didn't involve a whole lot of work and some guys told me about the trials studies. Went up there to GSK, I don't remember what it was for, something relatively benign. That first study was something like extra-strength Tylenol or something like that. They were looking at how long it would be in your bloodstream or something like that. It was pretty easy and I got paid all that money so I was, wow! I keep doing this, you know. For the first couple of years I don't think that I did any paid work at all. I only did clinical trials alone for two years because it was such a novelty, I could get money taking all these drugs. So, I did this for a couple of years, not doing nothing else, and then I started getting some more paid jobs occasionally but I kept doing the drug studies mostly at Jefferson. (Scott, 26 March 2004)

The anarchist community in West Philadelphia is concentrated around Baltimore Avenue from 45th Street to 49th and a few lateral streets on both sides of the avenue. It is a buffer zone between the gentrified areas adjacent to the University of Pennsylvania to the south, with remodeled houses and nicely kept apartments, and the dilapidated landscape of a lower-income African American community to the north. The neighborhood houses a vibrant community of immigrants from West Africa with food stores, restaurants, and shops. It also has a significant population of white, working-class and middle-class neighbors and a very vocal liberal community.

The visual signs of radical political activism are hard to miss. At 45th Street the local of the Industrial Workers of the World and the Communist Party league face each other, marking symbolically and physically the entrance into the area. Three blocks up, also on Baltimore and just next to the Dalhak, an Ethiopian bar, stands what local anarchists call "A Space," a hangout and organizing room identified by a big black sign with an encircled white capital "A" in the middle. A few houses away a colorful, hand-painted sign advertises the food co-op Mariposa, where most residents of the radical communal houses buy their food. On the corner of 50th Street and Baltimore stands the Firebird House, also a co-op, which repairs and sell bicycles. Bicycles play an important role in the community, enhancing the self-reliance and autonomy of their residents, who are able to circumvent the system by using a medium that is perceived to be not only cheaper than mass transit but also cleaner. Firebird House is also used by the community as a hangout where residents can exchange gossip and socialize; this is especially true during the summer, but community members ride their bicycles year-round. The Farm Market, next to Firebird House, provides fresh, organic vegetables to a community of politically engaged, hardcore vegans.

Twenty or thirty communal houses foster the anarchist community of the neighborhood. All the houses have names, such as Knot Squat (also known as "Not a Squat," after the occupants managed to buy the house from the city), Cider Garden, the Farm, Rainbow House, and House of the Future. At the corner of 49th Street was Fancy House, were I lived. Most of the houses have a porch filled with plants and sometimes objects that nobody cared to reclaim or remove. Although some of the fronts are painted, the houses all look somehow deliberately rough and unfinished. On the inside they are roomy, but even Fancy House, one of the best kept, had holes in the kitchen ceiling and the bathroom floor, no doubt a reflection of the owner's punk, hippie, and anarchist aesthetics and preferences. In addition to the residents' rooms, all the houses have a place for bicycles. Most backyards have a very well kept garden.

Fancy House is a good representative of the way the radical community organizes its housing arrangements in West Philadelphia. I moved there in early February 2004 and lived there until late August 2004. Although I knew Julie, its owner, I first had a meeting with the residents, who wanted to know if I could fit into their community. I had the credentials, was socially and politically aware, knew somebody in the house already, and was able to participate in "house meetings" and fulfill my assigned chores, which included emptying in the backyard garden the bucket with organic compost that we had in the kitchen. As in most community housing, residents of Fancy House cooked their meals together and wanted to know if I had a vegetarian diet. I didn't, but after I assured the residents that I was willing to contribute to the food expenses and would not use their pots to cook meat, they let me in. My presence helped to redress the gender imbalance at Fancy House. Finnley, in her mid-twenties, had arrived just a couple of months before I did and worked part-time at a magazine in Delaware. Marisa, also in her mid-twenties, had arrived from Kansas just a few weeks before Finnley and worked as a bike messenger. Asia, in her early thirties, was a close friend of Julie and was in a "sabbatical year" in New York. Asia had lived in the house for almost a year when I moved in and was a very active member of Act-Up. Jamie, in his mid-twenties, was also from Kansas and moved to Philadelphia at the same time Marisa did. He was also a bike messenger.

Michael, also in his twenties and also from Kansas, knew Marisa and Jamie before moving in. He was working in the kitchen of a catering firm when I moved and doing occasional clinical trials. The occupations of the Fancy House are typical of the radical West Philadelphia scene: the residents work in the informal economy, in badly paid jobs that do not have demanding schedules, leaving space for political and social activities. Other community members do paid community work as labor organizers or in community-based organizations such as Act-Up. Some radical community enterprises like Firehouse, the bicycle repair shop, or Wooden Shoe, the only anarchist library in the Philadelphia area, offer additional job possibilities in a cozy, community environment. At both locations men and women work equally and share profits in a cooperative arrangement, undisturbed by a loyal clientele that is not bothered by their display of long hair, bushy, nineteenth-century beards, tattoos, and piercings.

Living in community housing affords residents cheap rent and low food costs. Rent varied from $190 to $230 a month, depending on the size of the room. Every week $15 for food was deposited in a box kept in the fridge. The residents of Fancy House, like residents of almost all community housing in the neighborhood, shopped at the food co-op Mariposa, where every resident had to work two hours a month. Just a few weeks after I moved back to New York, Michael moved out of Fancy House, and in December, after saving enough "trial money," he flew to Spain.

The geographic mobility and instability among the residents of Fancy House reflect a larger trend among the radical community in West Philadelphia. Community members are always coming and leaving. In such a closely knit community, in which everyone knows everyone else, there is significant potential for disagreements and misunderstandings. This may explain why there is so much gossiping along with discussion of political and social issues. Members sometimes shift their social relationships by changing housing arrangements. If this is not enough, they may leave the city for a while for a similar community somewhere else. Networks connect anarchist communities in Seattle, Vermont, and West Virginia, among others.

"GUINEA-PIGGING" AS A LIFESTYLE

Ideology, community activism, lifestyle preferences, or just plain consumerism can induce volunteers to earn money only by participating in clinical trials, or to move back and forth between clinical trials and informal jobs. Like Scott, many professional guinea pigs feel attached to the novelty of selling their bodies as human subjects for toxicological clinical trials research. One guinea pig, Jennifer, described her year-and-a-half-long spree of participation by saying, "You become addicted to the easy money, you don't want to do anything else."

The paid volunteers whom I interviewed each participated in more than one trial. Some had volunteered for just a few, but most had been regular trial participants, with seven volunteers having done more than twenty phase I trials. Some remembered having done seventy, eighty, or even more, although they acknowledged losing track after a while. Eight volunteers had done between one and six trials, two volunteers between seven and thirteen, and one between fourteen and nineteen. Most of the volunteers surveyed had done at least one trial during the last year, many between two and five. Three volunteers had stopped participating in trials some years ago. Most of the participation took place in or around metropolitan Philadelphia.

The income derived from clinical trials allowed professional guinea pigs in the West Philly area to buy houses that they later transformed into communal housing, to travel around the world, to buy state-of-the-art computers, and to "chill." As noted above, trials afford volunteers flexible schedules and plenty of time to pursue other interests and occupations. While volunteers in the anarchist community of West Philadelphia pursued a broad range of activities and interests—as might be expected given the anarchist ethos of individuality—some general trends can be traced. For example, Dave Onion arrived in Philadelphia six years ago. A native of Washington State, he had lived as a child in the former Yugoslavia and later in Berlin, from where he traveled to Philadelphia, attracted by the possibility of living in an anarchist environment. There he learned about clinical trials, and after completing a few trials he was able to buy a dilapidated house from the City of Philadelphia for $5,000. Using his background as a construction worker, he rebuilt the property entirely, repairing roofs, refurbishing the kitchen, and installing solar panels to replace electric energy. The house has an unfinished, rough edge—even by community standards—and seems to be always undergoing some repair. The energy from the solar panels is not enough to support central heating or even a fridge, and the rooms have a gloomy, mysterious atmosphere. However, he has devised some ingenious methods to overcome these deficits. A wooden fireplace heats the kitchen, which is the social space of the house, and drinks can be cooled outside by placing them just behind the window in the winter. While Dave Onion's house is an extreme case of self-reliance and autonomy—other paid volunteers have chosen to make the commitment to a place and bought a house—it embodies the communitarian, anarchist ideal of living beyond a commodified, market-driven society.

Dave Onion used a considerable portion of his income to support the construction of a community space nearby. The space, a collective enterprise supported by other individuals and community organizations, was a half-finished building which progressed slowly because of the lack of steady investment. When completed it would accommodate Radio Volta, a community-based station transmitting from one of the communal houses in West Philadelphia. In addition, it will host a popular library (when I was there the books were still stored in boxes in the basement), a software and hardware computer training center for poor, mostly African American women (donated computer carcasses were piled up in a corner), and the office of the *Defenestrator*, an anarchist publication, among other projects.

Although the *Defenestrator* had an editorial board composed of Dave's girlfriend, Mc Mike (a veteran guinea pig and bike repair man at the Firehouse bike shop), and Paul (who also sat on the editorial board of the *Defenestrator*), among other occasional members, the publication was Dave Onion's brainchild. He wrote the majority of the articles, sold advertising space to friendly individuals and organizations, and contributed income from trials if needed. He also took charge of distribution, placing free copies at strategic places in the neighborhood like the A Space, the Food Market, Mariposa, and the Wooden Shoe bookstore. He was also involved in the Industrial Workers of the World (iww) and helped organize the annual commemoration of Worker's Day each May, usually a gathering in a nearby park accompanied by political discourses related to the occasion, workshops, music, food, and beverages.

The A Space provided a venue for political and community organizing. It was a center of antiwar activities, fundraisers, speeches in favor of the Chiapatistas movement and Guatemalan human rights, screenings of a documentary on worker-run factories in Argentina, and vegetarian dinners. In addition, it was at the A Space that Helms implemented the project "books behind bars," which collected books that he later delivered to prisoners in Pennsylvania. After he left for Paris a friend of his, a fellow professional guinea pig, continues Helms's work.

That anarchist members contributed books for this project reflects not only Helms's standing and reputation in the community but also the privileged position that literacy has among its members. Although their level of formal education is not particularly high, most residents have finished high school and a few others have some years of college or even a diploma, and reading and writing are a significant part of their everyday life. Many communal houses have libraries that include the classics of anarchist literature as well as works by García Márquez, Eduardo Galeano, and Noam Chomsky. Many residents work at the anarchist bookstore and have ready access to books and other printed materials. As noted above, the community has its own periodic publications, the *Defenestrator* and *Guinea Pig Zero*. Quite a few members explore different literary genres. Among volunteers, for example, Spam, an English major, writes short stories. The value accorded to literacy in this community is derived from their anarchist ethos, which accords a privileged position to self-education as a means of developing an alternative class understanding of the world based on the rejection of bourgeois values and practices. In addition, anarchist ideology also values the ability to work with one's own hands. Thus, it should come as no surprise that the anarchist community of West Philadelphia, and in particular its professional guinea pigs, should exhibit an enormous interest in developing some kind of craftsmanship, artisan work, or creative manual activity.

My roommate Michael was a professional jewelry and clothing designer who spent considerable time and effort working on his creations. Another volunteer plays the clarinet on Friday evenings at the local farmer's market. Volunteers at the Farm have converted the basement into a quasi-industrial carpentry site where they have created numerous wooden furniture pieces along with wood and metal sculptures. One of them also brews his own beer, which he stores in the basement.

Trial money also gives volunteers time to do community organizing. "The pharmaceutical industry is financing community activism in Philadelphia," said a close friend of Helms, the editor of *Guinea Pig Zero*. Almost all self-identified anarchist guinea pigs engaged in some kind of community activism, such as organizing International Workers' Day and rallies against the Iraq War, or working with Act-Up and other local community organizations. My fieldwork coincided with the beginning of the Iraq War, and this issue permeated not only my interactions with members of the community but also their everyday lives and organizing efforts. The community is intensely politicized, and local, national, and international politics were topics of animated debate.

Most clinical-trials volunteers are in their twenties and thirties, single, and childless, with flexible schedules and no permanent attachments.

Trial income offers them the opportunities to have fun and travel, and almost every weekend anarchists would hold elaborate parties in community houses that often included DJs and topical costumes. Sometimes they had a political or community fundraising purpose, but birthdays, Halloween, or just the welcome or farewell of a member of the community could serve as an excuse to socialize.

Radical guinea pigs also spend a significant amount of trial income on travel. Most volunteers have alternated periods of trial participation with extensive travel. Dave Onion traveled to Bulgaria, Mexico, and other destinations; Michael lived in Spain before coming to Philadelphia and left for Spain after completing a succession of trials; Spam had embarked on a tour that led him to South Asia and India; Helms had lived in France a few years ago and permanently resettled there a few months after I moved to Philadelphia.

In their spending habits guinea pigs show a clear understanding that their bodies are commodities, almost using their bodies as ATMs to fund their lifestyles. I discuss the commodification of the body in chapter 2.

KINGLABRAT

I met KingLabRat at the downtown youth hostel during my first reconnaissance trip to Philadelphia in the summer of 2002. Of Puerto Rican background, he alternated between Spanish and English while talking to me, mainly about women and sex, his most important concern aside from volunteering. KingLabRat was outspoken and talkative, not shy about being a professional guinea pig, and we readily formed a good bond. In his late thirties he had come from Florida for a trial at Wyeth, and in an effort to save money stayed for a few days at the hostel during the screening process and until he got admitted. Although we shared quite a bit of time together I did not carry out any formal observation then. When I returned to Philadelphia one year later I contacted him, and we made arrangements to meet when he was in the city for another trial. He arrived at the beginning of January from Wisconsin; he had tried to volunteer for a trial there, but things did not go as he had expected. After his arrival KingLabRat learned that the two-week trial, for which he was to be paid $3,000, would not start until one month later. For two weeks he stayed in a homeless shelter downtown, trying to hold out long enough to make it into the trial. KingLabRat explained to me that conditions at the shelter were bad and that he could not "take it anymore." He then traveled to Philadelphia by bus, arrived penniless, and, unable to afford even a cheap hotel, was staying with a Puerto Rican friend. He was hoping to enter a trial at GSK, pay some debts, and pocket some money.

I was able to go with KingLabRat through his trial at GSK. We met regularly before and after his screening, during the trial, and at the end. He was pleased with the attention and happy to help me with the research. When I suggested that he invent a pseudonym to protect himself against possible retaliation from the industry, he performatively chose to identify himself as KingLabRat. It suits him, since he is the most experienced professional guinea pig I have encountered. KingLabRat had been volunteering since he was discharged from the army in his early twenties for allegedly beating a sergeant. In between trials he sold drugs and worked in the morgue in Philadelphia. He had done trials since the mid-1980s at most of the trial facilities in the country from Miami to Texas, including the Midwest, and especially in New Jersey and Philadelphia. KingLabRat embodies—literally, in that his arms were covered by scars left by infinite needle punctures—the emergence of the market-recruited subject in pharmaceutical research. He provides a unique window into the way volunteers become professional guinea pigs.

KingLabRat's motivations to enter the trial are not different from those of the anarchist volunteers: the trials were a business, an opportunity to make money. But KingLabRat, unlike the anarchist volunteers, also believed that the trials offered an opportunity for scientific advancement. He told me: "We're doing something good for the people. Hey, the drug might work!" Whether other volunteers agreed or disagreed with KingLabRat on this score depended on how much credence they gave to the validity of scientific knowledge behind drug development. As we will see in chapters 1, 2, and 3, on major topics such as the social identity of paid subjects, the criteria for selecting trial subjects, and risk assessment and response, KingLabRat's positions do not differ in important aspects from those of the anarchist professional guinea pigs.

KingLabRat knew Helms and other regular anarchist subjects. He had volunteered with Helms at Wyeth a couple of years before, and when I asked about him, KingLabRat readily identified Helms as the "white guy." Racial differences were only part of KingLabRat's estrangement from Helms. KingLabRat was politically conservative, with a libertarian side, but this did not make him approve of the anarchist group. A devoted Catholic, he used to bring a bible to the trials, usually his only reading. According to him anarchism represented a totalitarian view that "imposed their ways of thinking on you." He elaborated this point: "atheists that shut down when you confront them. They don't like freethinkers." Emphatically, he noted that such an ideology is "wacky and politically wrong." Finally, he suggested that anarchism is "thievery," replacing private property by social property. In his current trial at GSK he had not encountered any anarchists.

During my first visit at the youth hostel I met another professional guinea pig. He was also in his thirties, white, from Canada, and had been living in the United States for a couple of years. Recently he had moved to Tennessee, where he hoped to launch a career as a folksinger, financing himself with the money earned as a volunteer. He encountered KingLab-Rat and used him to gain knowledge of the local trial scene. By chance, at the end of my fieldwork in July 2004 I stayed for a couple of days at the hostel and I was fortunate to find him again. He had come back to the city for a trial, also at GSK, so I followed him through.

KingLabRat and the Canadian guinea pig represent only a small portion of the universe of paid subjects volunteering in Philadelphia. While they share basic experiences and views with the radical anarchist volunteers, common to all paid subjects, they also have differences. The most important difference—besides the degree of altruism behind their participation—is their geographical mobility. Anarchist volunteers living in the West Philly community sometimes venture to trials in neighboring New Jersey and can eventually volunteer in trials in other areas. However, most of their trials are centered in the metropolitan Philadelphia region. By contrast, other professional guinea pigs—in particular those living outside Philadelphia—have greater mobility. One reason behind this difference is that Philadelphia affords enough trial opportunities to locals who do not need to travel beyond its limits. In addition, familiarity with social networks and trial facilities operates as a powerful incentive to volunteer in the area.

I do not want to overemphasize the lifestyle aspects behind guinea-pigging.

While for anarchists in West Philadelphia guinea pigging seems to be part of their lifestyle, for other groups or individuals beyond this enclave the aim of supporting a lifestyle may not be as strong, or may not be present at all. For some, joining trials is a way to pay increasing college costs, or gain some extra income in difficult times. But for the anarchists, entering the trial economy seems to be a calculated choice that provides income and the flexibility to pursue other interests. The industry's demands for flexible participants who can accommodate the schedules of clinical trials match the anarchists' desire for independence and autonomy. No wonder that most anarchists in Philadelphia had at one point or another joined the trial economy. They even developed a discourse to rationalize their trial participation. Not having a fixed, eight-hour schedule or a regular boss or employer also allows the anarchists to imagine that they are in some way "outside" the capitalist system. Of course, as I will argue in the Conclusion, they are not: they are a central component of drug development, fueling one of the most lucrative industries, and one with a global reach.

2

MARKET RECRUITMENT, IDENTITY, AND
RESISTANCE AMONG PROFESSIONAL GUINEA PIGS

"THE RENT-USE OF YOUR BODY AND THE INSIDE OPERATING FLUIDS"

When asked about what they think they are being compensated for as participants in a trial, volunteers do not hesitate. KingLabRat, a thirty-nine-year-old Latino volunteer who has traveled to almost every trial facility in the country since his early twenties and defines himself as a "professional lab rat," offers one of the most comprehensive answers: "It's for the rent-use of your body and the inside operating fluids; that's it pretty much in a nutshell." Paid volunteers understand that their body is a commodity and that it is for their body that they are being "compensated" by the pharmaceutical industry. Hinting at the alienation produced by volunteering in paid clinical-trials research, Helms noted that "they don't care about your mind, they want you for your body."

As seen in chapter 1, volunteers participate in trials strategically, to support themselves or their lifestyles. Volunteers' clear understanding of their bodies as a commodity stands in opposition to the industry's denial that commodification is taking place. The industry uses a series of rhetorical moves to disclaim its reliance on commoditized bodies. One is the industry's definition of "paid volunteers" who receive "financial compensation for time and travel expenses." It is hard not to note the oxymoron. How can someone simultaneously be paid to do something and do it voluntarily?

In fact the volunteers are workers who place their bodies and their time at the service of the pharmaceutical industry, but by denying that labor is being extracted the industry intends to place the "exchange" beyond the reach of labor laws. Yet even as the industry seeks to deny commodification through a language that stresses voluntariness, and avoids references to labor, pain, and suffering, it contradicts itself by offering easy money to volunteers who otherwise would have no motivation to participate. The volunteers are quick to note the cynicism of the industry's approach. They realize that their participation is not free of constraints, and that it is money that induces them to participate in research trials. This point will be further explored in chapter 7 in relation to volunteers' perception of the informed-consent process.

Professional guinea pigs understand that when they volunteer in a trial they are entering a contractual business relationship. Some volunteers explicitly defined their work status as "short-term contractors," having signed a contract and an informed-consent form that refers to specific duties, responsibilities, rights, and even the obligation to pay taxes (although this is a mere formality, since most volunteers never consider doing so).

THE MILD TORTURE ECONOMY: "YOU ARE NOT ASKED TO PRODUCE OR TO DO SOMETHING ANYMORE, YOU ARE BEING ASKED TO ENDURE SOMETHING"

Volunteers understand their participation as trial subjects as a particular type of work not based on physical labor—the traditional image of work and workers, influenced by their anarchist and working-class background. Professional guinea pigs have the sense that while volunteering for a trial they do not do much except just lie there—or, as Frank Little put it in chapter 1, "except for the needles and the pills it sounds like a vacation." Most guinea pigs would agree with Spam, who was quoted in the Introduction as describing the trials as "a weird type of work" in a "mild torture economy," in which one is paid not to produce something but "to endure" something, while subjecting oneself to regimes of science and capital accumulation.

Most of the time that volunteers spend as inpatients is filled with dead periods when they are just lying in bed, waiting to do a blood draw, or just hanging around chatting, watching TV, playing games, or reading. Like the security guard from Spam's example, volunteers are bored most of the time, and this is one of their main complaints about the experience of being a guinea pig. In addition, volunteering can be painful, in particular if the blood draws are not performed skillfully or if there is trouble finding a vein, which are common occurrences. KingLabRat boasted about his capacity to tolerate pain, which he saw as a sign of his masculinity. He also confided to me how he dealt with the discomforts of being a research subject. He said that he focuses not on his body and what is going on. Instead he thinks about the things he will do with the money he receives. The detachment between the mind and the body experiences and the emphasis on material gains and planning are similar to the strategies adopted by sex workers during sexual encounters.

The understanding that their body is a commodity and that they are entering a market transaction also shapes the volunteers' social identity. Rejecting the industry notion of "paid volunteers," participants who derive their main income from clinical trials, and long-time veterans of trials, usually identify themselves as professional guinea pigs. Volunteers coined the verb "guinea pigging" to define their professional activity.

> Well, not "patient," because this would imply that they are doing something to improve your health. Kind of worker, although such a strange kind of work, definitely guinea pig. Well, I think that it's both, worker and guinea pig because you are paid to take this risk and also for this kind of weird dehumanization. It's funny, what gets me the most is getting EKGs, I guess. And it's funny because it's for my safety and it is not invasive, has no side effects, but I take my clothes off and these people start putting things over my naked chest and then is when I feel like a guinea pig more than a worker. It's so much like sex work, like being exposed to a dominatrix out there, it's so demanding. It's something that most people wouldn't get through. The guinea pig part is also because they pay you just to demean you to animal status, you are just letting yourself be measured by the functions of your organs and stuff, something that most people wouldn't agree with. (Shon, 12 June 2004)

It is clear that human volunteers are guinea pigs only in a figurative, metaphorical sense. Analyzing these metaphors is important because they shed light on the relationship between paid volunteers and the pharmaceutical industry. They are also key to understanding social identity among guinea pigs, and the relationship that they enter into when they volunteer for a trial. The metaphor of the professional guinea pig encapsulates the identity of workers who have a profession or trade, and those who are paid to take risks and be dehumanized. Shon's definition of the guinea pig evokes the image of the animal traditionally used in biomedical research, an animal associated with passivity, objectification, and ultimately alienation, and his association of professional guinea pigs with sex workers is made frequently among professional guinea pigs. Echoing Spam's idea that volunteers are paid to "endure something" in a "mild torture" economy, Helms elaborates: "There are similarities with sex work because you get penetrated, you get needles, you get the tubes, whatever. They are penetrating your body. You really get penetrated. It is not an illusion; it is not a figurative thing. That's one similarity with the sex work. Another thing is that you are renting up your body and they don't care about what you are thinking and they don't want to be talked about, they just want your body to do something and react to the drug so they can watch it" (Helms, 15 January 2005).

There is another connotation of the term "guinea pig": the taking of risks in an experimental context where the outcomes are uncertain. Volunteers are aware of the ethical violations, human rights abuses, and even horror of biomedical research. (How much they know about the risks they face and how they respond to them will be the topic of chapter 3.) Professional guinea pigs, unlike other workers, do not sell their labor power every day in a continuous relationship. Instead a guinea pig sells his or her services in a discrete way based on a fragmented trial participation. Paid volunteers are contractors who shift from one trial to another, alternating with periods of working at other informal jobs or just plain unemployment.

In the view of the guinea pigs, the payment received is not for abstract "time" as measured by the pharmaceutical industry, but instead for the time filled with boredom and the discomfort experienced during the trial. The industry may recognize this, since the amount of money that volunteers receive is related to the discomfort of the procedures, such as the number of blood extractions, intubations, or more invasive procedures, as well as the time spent in the trials. Professional guinea pigs are familiar with these criteria, and experienced guinea pigs boast that they can predict the amount of money they will receive for a trial based on a specified schedule and procedures.

The short-term nature of engagement with a research site has serious consequences for the way guinea pigs see long-term risks. Once the trial is over volunteers tend to think that the risk is also over. Unlike miners and other workers who are exposed to hazardous substances, the guinea pigs lack the social networks and shared experiences that would allow them to focus on long-term risks. While anarchist volunteers form a more stable and closely knit community than other paid subjects, the observation still holds. (I develop this theme in my discussion of risk in chapter 3.)

GUINEA PIG ZERO

As E. P. Thompson has shown in *The Making of the English Working Class*, the production of print materials helped to shape the class identity of the eighteenth-century English working class. In this masterpiece Thompson demonstrates how through the production, distribution, and discussion of journals, pamphlets, and other documents, industrial workers come to reflect and shape their identity as a group of people with similar interests, opposed to the interests of the capitalist class. Guinea pigs have also employed journals to nurture forms of professional identification and solidarity, enabling them to form a common identity based on their experiences. They also display similar forms of knowledge that include medical lingo and humor, and they share a working-class identification, perhaps unsurprisingly since most professional guinea pigs hold working-class jobs.

Guinea Pig Zero: A Journal for Human Research Subjects was edited in Philadelphia by Robert Helms from 1996 to 2000, during which eight issues were published. The first issues were sold for $2, although later issues which included more pages were sold for slightly more. Back issues could also be purchased for $4. Estimates about readership are hard to make because the editor kept printing and selling old issues by request along with recent ones, but he places its reach between five hundred and a thousand. In 2002, after discontinuing the zine, the editor decided to publish an anthology of *Guinea Pig Zero*.

Although Helms wrote and edited most of the contents of the zine, he saw *Guinea Pig Zero* as the product of the collective efforts of professional guinea pigs across the country. "I tried to portray the experiences not only of myself but other guinea pigs I knew and knew about GPZ. In particular places I also give my own opinion but it was me based on a group of people who had done it. It wasn't just based on my own experience and nothing else." The zine, according to its editor, was a forum to voice the "perspective of the guinea pigs and that's all it ever tried to be. The company can go to hell. They are not writing this magazine."

Helms decided to publish a zine just a few months after he started doing clinical trials. Before entering trials he majored in classical studies at Temple University, where he also participated in student protests in support of the striking faculty. Later he took a job as a field organizer for the Hospital Worker's Union. From 1991 to 1994 he spent time campaigning with human service workers. After he left his last job he worked at painting, carpentering, and construction jobs in Philadelphia. Although he entered his first trial in the mid-1990s and kept volunteering until he left for France in 2003, he also kept doing some work on the side to supplement his trial income. He does not remember exactly how many trials he has done, but they number more than eighty, at least half of them at Jefferson Hospital, the only place that allowed Helms to take part in trials after he became well known for editing GPZ.

Helms based his journal on earlier models like *Dishwasher* and *Temp Slave!* Both belong to a subgenre known as the jobzine, which according to Helms "treated unglamorous jobs as the platforms of culture" (Helms 2002). In a personal interview he expanded his understanding of the genre. "[A jobzine] is a zine about what people would consider a crummy job, not a career goal and not having a career goal that necessary goes farther than that. In other words, you had a life but your life was not around working for somebody else, your psychology was not sold out, you had your own identity. Your world did not include what your boss said your world was. Your work was just your work, you were yourself, your own person and your goal was not to kiss your boss's ass. Labor movement kind of idea, job zine with emphasis in a particular trade and also the idea of freedom from industry. I never took an ad" (Helms, 15 January 2005).

The first issue, thirty-two pages long and in black and white, was published on 1 May 1996. The cover inaugurated a tradition by depicting a guinea pig wearing a hat and tie. Later issues would depict guinea pigs attached to medical instruments, lying dead, or standing on a bowl supposedly containing Paxil, a psychiatric drug. The date chosen for publication of the first issue, celebrating a major landmark in labor organizing and identity, was deliberate, although the magazine itself did not make any explicit reference to it. While Helms did not hide his anarchist beliefs he chose not to make his political ideology the center of the zine, which nevertheless was clearly focused on the working class, labor issues, and guinea pig identity and solidarity.

The introductory editorial of *Guinea Pig Zero* presented the zine as a space in which to discuss experiences from a guinea pig's perspective. The point was that in contrast to the objectifying, alienating treatment that guinea pigs receive as research subjects, they are mindful subjects with shared trajectories and interests: "[Scientists] want us to tell them how we're feeling, and whether our minds and bodies are coming apart, and then to leave it at that. But every guinea pig discovers, after a short period of time with the species, that we constantly tell each other what's on our minds. In fact, we have a little society of our own, with folklore, our own strange humor, special cares and most importantly, a commonality of interests" (Helms 2002). The publication stressed that the interests of guinea pigs stood in opposition to those of the scientific establishment and in particular the pharmaceutical industry. According to Helms's editorial, it is "unnatural for a guinea pig to let the scientists know what he's thinking."

One of the goals of *Guinea Pig Zero* was to rescue the value of the contribution that human subjects made to further biomedical research. While volunteering for a trial might be alienating and dehumanizing, according to Helms "on the other hand it takes the human research subject to the level of civilization when he or she looks in the mirror and sees the face of a specialized worker, whose craft has its own wondrous history, its own jargon and its own little culture" (Helms 2002). This proud identification of guinea pigs with their work no doubt echoes the way workers have spoken about themselves since the beginning of the industrial revolution.

The first issue of *Guinea Pig Zero* provides a glimpse into guinea pig history. One of the main concerns of the zine was the radical reappropriation of the history of human subjects in experimental research. According to the standard narrative, biomedical science was at the center with volunteers at the margin. The first article in the zine, "The Treadmill of History," explored the history of human participation in biomedical experimentation, stressing the contributions made by volunteers and the ethical violations of their rights. There were also sections on guinea pig humor, home remedies offering help "for clean, fresh blood," and a review of *The Double Blind*, a novel involving clinical trials written in the 1960s by John Rowan Wilson.

Later issues of the zine reveal a preoccupation with revalorizing the contribution of human subjects to biomedical research throughout history, and attempts to foster a guinea pig "culture" with shared meanings, interpretations, and forms of humor. One issue offered humorous hints in an item entitled "How You Will Know That's He's a Pro: The Signs of a Bona Fide Guinea Pig." Among the clues: wearing clothing or accessories printed with the research unit's logos; knowing more about blood chemistry than a second-year medical student; interrogating waitresses about the poppy seed content of bread products; and referring to one's anticubital vein as a "financial pipeline." It is easy to see the pride in being a professional guinea pig in these jokes. Other jokes I heard during my fieldwork make the same point by stressing and ridiculing the differences between a professional guinea pig and an inexperienced, paid human subject.

The second issue of *Guinea Pig Zero* introduced report cards summarizing professional guinea pigs' evaluations of clinical facilities throughout the country. Grades were given for the average amount of compensation per study, the quality of the facilities and the food provided during the trials, the professionalism and skills of the staff, the absence of unnecessary procedures during the screening process and changes in the schedule, and subjective factors such as the environment of the research facility. Since the evaluations depended on accounts by individual guinea pigs, some were more detailed than others, although all covered what were regarded as the important points to consider in choosing a research facility.

The report cards were one of the more popular sections of the zine and represented Helms's attempt to stress shared material interests among professional guinea pigs. While other sections of the zine challenged dominant representations of guinea pigs among the biomedical sector, the report cards signaled a more direct threat that could interfere with the capacity of such places to recruit new human subjects. If the facility was a contract research organization (CRO) hired by a pharmaceutical company to conduct trials, a bad grade could also alert the sponsor of the trial to review the contract with the organization. It is not surprising that after *Harper's* republished one of the report cards from *Guinea Pig Zero* that reported the failures of a clinical trial research facility, Helms was sued for libel.

Although the case was dismissed, the emotional drain of facing a trial and what Helms called an act of "cowardice" by *Harper's* when it printed a partial retraction left him wary. Entering the debate about the libel lawsuit, *Philadelphia Magazine* confirmed independently that the report card issued by *Guinea Pig Zero* was accurate. Helms covered the libel suit in *Guinea Pig Zero*, providing a class analysis to explain how the publisher of *Harper's*, grandson of the billionaire philanthropist John D. MacArthur, sided with the interests of the industry and against *Guinea Pig Zero*. This episode also served as a cautionary tale for me, by alerting me to the potential conflicts that might arise from the critique of a very powerful industry.

THE GUINEA PIGS REVOLT

In December 2002 a group of guinea pigs volunteering for a study at Jefferson successfully challenged a major pharmaceutical company and obtained a significant concession by threatening to walk out in the middle of the trial. When I met Helms a few months later, one of the first things he asked me was if I was familiar with the strike at Jefferson. Dave Onion, a close friend of Helms and also a veteran guinea pig living in West Philly, had joined the same trial and gave his version of the event in the *Defenestrator*, an occasional publication that represents the views of the anarchist community in Philadelphia. Helms also wrote a piece for the Industrial Workers of the World (iww), an anarcho-syndicalist union. Every guinea pig in West Philly was familiar in one way or another with the walkout at Jefferson and offered his or her candid perspectives on it. Even guinea pigs who were not in the area at the time and who moved into the city later on soon became socialized into the master strike narrative. Part of their excitement, no doubt, was due to the success that the guinea pigs had in challenging a powerful company for which they had no sympathy. The event was the first time that guinea pigs in the West Philadelphia radical scene had successfully used the threat of a walkout to press the pharmaceutical industry to accept their demands.

The trial started in early December at the facilities of Jefferson, a research hospital of one of the oldest and more traditional medical schools in the city. Volunteers tested a low dose of an anti-anxiety drug—"enough to cause some drowsiness but too low for a mood change," according to Helms—for a major pharmaceutical company that regularly carries out its phase I clinical trials at this facility. The trial, including pre-screenings and follow-up appointments, lasted seven weeks. According to the schedule the trial would have five stages in which volunteers were supposed to stay in the hospital for four days, with thirty-six-hour releases between the stages and a break for Christmas and New Year's. As is typical for extended trials involving invasive or unusual procedures, the recruiters selected experienced, reliable guinea pigs. Among the volunteers there was a slight majority of African Americans, followed by white volunteers, all between the ages of eighteen and forty-five, the usual age range in phase I clinical trials research. Three volunteers were from the radical West Philadelphia scene and most volunteers knew each other from earlier studies.

As part of the trial subjects had to defecate in a container so that the staff could search for the remains of the drug tablet. Along with this procedure, a catheter was inserted and fifteen blood samples were collected during each stage. The volunteers' diet was regulated so that all would get the same meals. For the duration of the trial volunteers were required to abstain from drinking alcohol or using any other drug, including aspirin or vitamins.

Volunteers were to receive $3,350 for completion of the study. Before the first stage was over everyone agreed that the pay was too low for the inconveniences caused by the trial's schedule. Guinea pigs were talking about leaving for better-paying trials in the area and complaining about the conditions of the trial. In particular, the impossibility of drinking alcohol during the Christmas break caused major worries among volunteers. Dave Onion summarized their mood: "I think that it was really a collective thing. And it is not always that people start talking about leaving. There were many folks saying: 'I'm getting the fuck out of here and I am gonna screen for this other study.' Especially because it was Christmas it was a lot of people willing to lose the $1,000 they would get for finishing the second part of the trial, you know. And also, it was such a pain in the ass to do the study: it was not like you could go, sit down and read a book or anything. You were constantly being demanded to do something else every twenty minutes or something. It just like made sense to us to do something like that" (Dave Onion, 18 May 2004).

A few days into the study volunteers asked Helms to write a one-page memorandum that "respectfully" asking for financial compensation to be increased to $4,500. Helms was well known both to volunteers and to the staff at Jefferson, which he had earlier evaluated for *Guinea Pig Zero*, giving it credit for decent pay and professionalism. However, he took care not to appear to be the organizer of the event. When gathering signatures for the memorandum he was careful to show that the argument was not coming mainly from him. "Another guinea pig walked the paper around the ward in plain view of the staff and I signed my name in the middle of the list rather than first," he confided. Within a day volunteers managed to secure the signatures of all but one volunteer. However, there was peer pressure on this last holdout after the list was completed, and he asked the management to let him sign it too. Six volunteers met the staff to formally deliver their memorandum with their claims.

To influence management, volunteers kept talking among themselves about leaving the study in the middle for other studies, which would have caused a major financial setback to the sponsor since all the data collected to that time would have become useless. On the other hand, quitting a trial after the first half is over deprives a volunteer of half his income, which is prorated. Helms suggested that volunteers ingest flexible vinyl propaganda scraps, so that the staff would find little notes reading "more money" in their feces, but his idea was rejected.

After delivering their note, the volunteers were promised an answer before the holiday break. Trial managers informally assured the volunteers that they understood and agreed with their request. The final decision, though, rested with the pharmaceutical industry that sponsored the trial and paid the expenses. On the evening before the volunteers were about to leave for the holiday break they had not heard from management and were increasingly anxious about their demands. Just a few hours before their release, the unit director summoned all volunteers to the lounge for a brief announcement. Jefferson had got authorization from the sponsor to raise the financial compensation. Instead of the sum requested in their memo guinea pigs received an additional $800, which was still "plenty of money." The volunteers "cheered and thanked [the staff] profusely," Helms wrote. Before the meeting broke, the nurse "emphatically stated" that what happened should not set a precedent and that volunteers could not "band together" to put pressure on a sponsor in the middle of a trial. She assumed that this was an unusual case, where the financial compensation had not taken the special trial requirements into account.

According to written and oral testimonies by Helms and Dave Onion of the successful walkout, the event erupted almost spontaneously, without major organizational work. While anarchist guinea pigs certainly played a role in the events, they are quick to emphasize that they were not instrumental in leading it. "Some people had some union background and I was surprised how easy it was. I know some union organizers, and just watching them trying to organize people, even on a small scale, it's not easy for them. For us it was just little effort, like two people needed some work but everybody else was on board from the beginning" (Dave Onion, 18 May 2004).

While the walkout was a collective enterprise, this should not obscure the role played by more radical guinea pigs in articulating demands and presenting them to the staff. Helms, with his experience as a labor organizer and his familiarity with the staff, played a key role in efforts to mobilize guinea pigs. This was also his last trial. He was soon to reach forty-five years of age, the limit for phase I volunteers. The displeasure among volunteers with what they thought were unfair clinical-trial conditions might have provided him with an opportunity to finally fight the pharmaceutical industry.

The confluence of radical labor organizers and a population of professional guinea pigs volunteering for a trial under unfair or tough labor conditions has no doubt presented itself before, if not in other cities then at least in the Philadelphia area. Why did it take so long to successfully launch a concerted collective effort to address these problems? And what does this successful attempt mean for the guinea pigs and the pharmaceutical industry conducting clinical trials in the region?

While open conflict between volunteers and staff is rare, the potential for more veiled forms of conflict between staff and volunteers is embedded in the social organization of the trial. Members of the staff such as nurses, technicians, and lower-ranking administrators and recruiters are the first to mediate between management and volunteers. This buffer position exposes them to the demands, concerns, and anxieties of the volunteers. Male anarchists tend to be more sympathetic than other volunteers toward nurses. Anarchist volunteers tend to see registered nurses, phlebotomists, and other technicians on the staff as occupying low-paying jobs which are also exploited forms of labor. Certainly this sympathy does not prevent them from complaining when they think that the staff lacks skill. In particular, poor blood extractions have painful consequences for volunteers, who are sometimes not shy about their discomfort.

There are also other problems. Changes in schedule cause major inconveniences for guinea pigs by altering their schedules and disrupting their work, political and social activities, and social life. African American and Latino volunteers can experience discriminatory treatment. KingLabRat felt clearly that race was an issue in the way the staff related to him and others, an impression that I was able to confirm by talking with radical white male volunteers. Since I was unable to observe directly the relationships between staff and volunteers, or among volunteers themselves, I had to rely on indirect accounts through the narratives of the volunteers.

In addition to these structural sources of conflict, the threatened walkout was a collective response prompted by what volunteers perceived as unfair and unusual working conditions. While bad or just plain hospital foods or excessive blood draws are present in many clinical trials, the need to preserve feces is not a usual arrangement. According to Helms, volunteers were unhappy about the odors and discomfort caused by the procedure. Still, what gave them the sense that the trial conditions were too hard or intolerable for the amount of money they would receive was that the trial schedule had been changed since it was signed by volunteers, and it was so compressed that as Helms put it, "practically you had no wash out periods [breaks], you were always in the trial."

As a result of the changes, the trial, which was supposed to be conducted during the fall, was pushed up to the last weeks of the year and extending past New Year's Eve. When the volunteers started the trial they soon realized that they would need to come back after the Christmas break for the last part of the trial. This realization, along with the organizational efforts of savvy anarchist organizers among them, who rallied volunteers to sign the memo, might have been enough to successfully launch the walkout threat.

According to Helms and Onion, one of the conditions that made the event a success was that all the volunteers were professional guinea pigs who knew each other from the trials. Two central conditions were thus instrumental in launching the walkout threat. Being professional volunteers, members had a shared understanding of what it was possible to accomplish in the context of a clinical trial. They knew that their numbers and the structure of the trial, divided into many "legs," afforded them a relatively powerful position. If the trial could not be continued the sponsor would both lose all the data and have its research schedule seriously compromised. A professional body of volunteers also ensured that there would be sufficient mutual trust to engage in such an event. As Helms told me, "Nobody is gonna risk their money for somebody they don't know and that they don't trust."

Another strength of the effort was its focus on a single, central, and immediate demand: an increase in the amount of money paid for the clinical trial. The guinea pigs did not attempt to change working conditions permanently, or to address larger issues related to the way clinical trials are organized and conducted. The volunteers were clear in limiting their grievances to one trial and its special circumstances. Despite the differences among volunteers, they all shared an interest in maximizing their income. Although this contributed to their success, it did not provide grounds for extending their collective action beyond immediate material concerns. "I also think that what happened at Jefferson was in part, a unique situation. I think that it will be difficult to organize guinea pigs because so many people are coming and going, there is a lot of instability with people that are guinea pigs too. Half of the people are just doing it for once or twice and it would be difficult to make them take a bit of a risk. They just want to get some easy dollars and don't think about it again. I think that it might be easier to get people together around other issues around safety, accountability and health kind of stuff. I think that's what worries people more" (Dave Onion, 18 May 2004).

According to Helms and Onion, but also many other guinea pigs whom I interviewed, working conditions are usually good at Jefferson. As mentioned earlier, Helms gave the facility unusually high grades in his ranking of clinical-trial research sites, emphasizing the staff's professionalism and recognizing the pay scale as standard for the industry. Given the comparatively high income afforded by volunteering in clinical trials, participants have few incentives to challenge the industry.

Another possible explanation for the difficulty in organizing guinea pigs is they are a very mobile and unstable population. Some guinea pigs travel across the country seeking the most profitable trial opportunities. In addition, volunteers move in and out of clinical trials, alternating their work in trials with other activities. To complicate things more, clinical trials can last as little as two or three inpatient days, and seldom last more than a few weeks. After the trial ends the volunteers may not see each other for a long time, if ever.

All the informants whom I talked to about the possibilities for an organized guinea pig action suggested that it was very unlikely to happen under the current circumstances. The capitalist system needed to change before we could see a union of guinea pigs, they noted, and that seemed unlikely given the conservative and anti-union mood of the country.

An awareness of the limits for any kind of sustained organizational work among guinea pigs dampened their excitement about the success of the walkout. Helms edited an anthology of *Guinea Pig Zero* for a popular press and discontinued publication of the magazine. Just a few months after his last trial participation at Jefferson he moved to France, where he took up residence in a working-class neighborhood in the suburbs of Paris. He gained his living by doing some painting and construction jobs, although his difficulty with the French language made things hard for him. He was considering doing some clinical trials in Paris as well.

It is also difficult to forecast how the successful walkout might shape the organization of future clinical trials in the area. After participating in the walkout Onion did a couple of trials, although not at this facility. He was unsure about how the pharmaceutical industry might respond to the walkout, but hinted at the possibility that they might end up moving south, where labor costs were lower and organized opposition less likely. "I am sure Merck thought about it too but I am not totally sure which effect it had in reality. I think that a lot of studies are apparently moving south. I think that Merck or some big pharmaceutical company just opened a place in the South. The North people are paid a lot more than in the South. I've heard about some places in the South that you get paid $100 a day or $150 a day. Compare that to [Bristol Meyers], which for some studies is paying $400 a day. I think that for the pharmaceutical industry, companies like Merck that should sound a red light in the sense that they have to improve things if they don't want to lose trials patients to the South or whatever. I don't know: it's hard to tell, really" (Dave Onion, 18 May 2004).

The landscape of the pharmaceutical industry in Philadelphia changed dramatically almost two years after the events of December 2002. Merck, the pharmaceutical giant that sponsored clinical-trial research at Jefferson, ran into serious trouble when its billion-dollar blockbuster drug

Vioxx was retired from the market after the FDA announced that it presented an unacceptable risk for patients. While there are still trials being conducted at Jefferson, its operations as a CRO seem to be affected at least temporarily by Merck's troubles. In addition, GSK, another international pharmaceutical company based in the city, announced recently that it has stopped its recruitment of phase I volunteers. I am not suggesting that these developments are related to the successful walkout threat at Jefferson. They seem to be the product of international, national, and local considerations. What is certain, however, is that these events have the potential to alter radically the livelihoods of hundreds or thousands of people who in one way or another relied on the income provided by participation in clinical trials.

TRIAL DISRUPTIONS

While organized forms of collective action against pharmaceutical industry interests are rare among volunteers, individual acts of resistance, or what de Certau called "resistance of the weak" (de Certau 1982), plague the routine development of clinical trials. Professional guinea pigs have a number of ways of resisting or challenging the authority and power embedded in the organization of trials, obliquely and indirectly.

For example, professional guinea pigs consciously attempt to disrupt the way clinical trials are organized. Usually the food provided during inpatient trials is at best institutional food, homogeneous and not very tasty. This circumstance provides the guinea pigs with a good excuse to supplement their diet as inpatients with food sneaked in from outside. Clinical-trial settings vary in how stringently they search volunteers who enter a trial facility as subjects. Most research sites in the Philadelphia area do not do so. The preferred contraband items of professional guinea pigs include seeds, peanuts, and fruit. Most volunteers are not vegetarians—in theory vegetarians are excluded from clinical trials—but some vegetarians lie so that they can be admitted, and once in a trial they find it hard to follow a meat-based diet. Except in the few trials where the staff closely monitors the dietary intake of volunteers, undercover vegetarians trade food with others, exchanging meat for vegetables.

Avoiding a trial's drug is not possible for inpatient volunteers, who are closely monitored, but outpatient trials are less strict and have fewer means of ensuring compliance. During fieldwork I met some outpatient

volunteers who avoided taking part of the drug or drug regimen, sometimes doing so individually and at other times coordinating their noncompliance with other volunteers. This sort of noncompliance could be
opportunistic, when controls were lax or nonexistent, or it could be a
rebellious act, particularly among anarchist professional guinea pigs who
hold a clear anti-industry stand. Shon, an anarchist volunteer with more
than ten years of experience in paid clinical trials, is not shy about
explaining his attempts to resist and subvert everyday routines when he
was a human subject: "I even try to sabotage the results now and then. I
am pretty cynical and don't think that the trials result in much medical
benefit and most of the guinea pigs feel just the same way. So we bring in
snacks when we are supposed to be fasting. I do it consciously to screw
them, but other people do it because they are veggies and are hungry and
in part to screw them and take their dignity back. It's a pretty common
thing that people are always bringing things in and it really fucks up the
data, you know. If you are going to do a blood test and you just had a
candy bar before, that would bust your sugar levels a lot. But, so, I don't
have any bad conscience about perpetuating capitalism by being exploited by the pharmaceutical industry" (Shon, 12 June 2004).

Shon is not alone in his cynicism. Anarchist volunteers do not have
faith in clinical-trials research and the pharmaceutical industry. Industry
and government pretend, contrary to the evidence, that the demands for
a perfectly healthy volunteer can be met. In addition, the sense among
anarchist subjects that women and minorities are excluded from clinical
trials, possibly skewing the outcomes, adds to their cynicism. And apart
from their lack of belief in the promises of science, anarchist volunteers
share an opposition to a process that exploits and dehumanizes volunteers. Small acts of resistance are a way to recover their humanity and
agency when faced with a powerful institution and a social system that
they oppose.

Regardless of what some of the anarchist volunteers may believe, their
perceived acts of disruption and sabotage do not challenge the outcome of
the trials. Mindful of these acts of resistance, organizers of clinical trials
create a controlled setting, with heavy surveillance of volunteer's bodies,
dose intake, and diet. I believe that if anything threatens the validity of
clinical-trials research it is not the limited attempts by volunteers to
disrupt the process but rather the lack of representation of women and

other demographic groups in phase I trials, statistical manipulation that makes outcomes appear significant when they might not be clinically relevant, and, worst of all, the hiring of ghostwriters and paid "consultants" to interpret and present data in a favorable light during later phases of drug development (Angell 2004). In addition, as I will argue later, the main problem with most phase I drug trials is not their lack of validity but their lack of innovation, since most are trials for me-too drugs, which resemble drugs already in the market but which in the view of the companies can be a profitable new version of the same thing.

In light of the cynical view that anarchist volunteers have of clinical trials and their traditional hostility toward the pharmaceutical industry, how do they explain to themselves their engagement as clinical-trial subjects, which may benefit the industry they despise? Radical male professional guinea pigs do not see their participation in a trial as a contradiction. They have thought about this issue, and their narrative is very uniform and carefully laid out. They point out that both the pharmaceutical industry and they themselves intend to make money performing clinical-trials research. In their view, exploitation is inalienable in the capitalist society, and dependent labor relationships will be exploitative as long as they remain in the capitalist framework. Working for the pharmaceutical industry may be exploitative, but the same was true of their jobs driving trucks, making fast food, or sorting packages on a conveyor belt.

"FARMGIRL": FEMALE PAID SUBJECTS

While I met fewer anarchist women in my fieldwork I cannot avoid noting that those whom I did meet seemed to be as critical of the pharmaceutical industry as their male counterparts, but also more troubled by their role as subjects. Farmgirl, in her mid-twenties, had moved from Chicago to Philadelphia less than two years earlier, lived in a couple of houses in the West Philly community, and earned her income doing trials research and working part-time as an office cleaner. She regularly sold her blood for $70 until she learned about the possibility of volunteering for the more lucrative inpatient trials. She had done five trials, almost exclusively at Jefferson. Farmgirl, who does not take medicines in her everyday life and has participated in campaigns against pharmaceutical companies, is troubled by her role as a subject:

Definitely it actually makes me sick that [the pharmaceutical companies] rub the money in front of my face and I take it and support something that I don't support in any other way and don't want to support. It is also something that is kind of easy to justify. When I did the first study it was just because I didn't have any money. And I justified it like: this is a part of society I don't believe in and do not want to be a part of, and here I am, and poor me. Of course, I take money from the drug companies because they suck, I take their money. But now I have more money and feel that I cannot do it any more, at all. Maybe I take a break but then they call you and tell you "just come for five minutes and get $1,000,000." And once you do them it is kind of addictive, you just keep doing it. But I definitely hate these companies. I have spent time boycotting Procter and Gamble and other companies and then these pharmaceuticals offer you all this money and here I am, back again. I hate them, really hate them. It is something I definitely struggle with. (Farmgirl, 1 June 2004)

Women, like their anarchist male counterparts, are quick to express their antipathy toward the pharmaceutical industry and the state, and their mistrust of them. But anarchist women are more likely to acknowledge that their participation in clinical trials is a contradiction, because it helps the pharmaceutical industry's profits and represents a biomedical model based on treatment rather than prevention, of which they are also very critical. This is an important distinction. Although male professional guinea pigs are critical of the ethics of biomedical research, they are less vocal about the science behind the trials. This fact has a direct relevance to the way professional guinea pigs understand and deal with the risks they face as clinical-trial subjects. (This is the topic of chapter 3.)

As mentioned earlier, women have fewer opportunities to participate in trials and usually do not rely on them as their main source of income. Anarchist women have only sporadic possibilities of entering the trial economy, and therefore they are freer than their male counterparts to take a tougher stand toward the pharmaceutical industry and the social organization of trials research.

3

LOCAL KNOWLEDGE AND RISK MANAGEMENT
AMONG PROFESSIONAL GUINEA PIGS

> So you know, when you start doing studies you start meeting the regulars
> that have been doing trials frequently, maybe ten years if not longer, and
> they are fine. You hear from time to time some horror stories but they seem
> to be such an exception. So when I talk with people that have been doing it
> for a very long time I think that trials are really very low-risk compared to
> these other occupations I was talking about. But there are a few things that
> make me wonder. I've noticed that people sometimes, maybe because they
> are scared to think about it, don't really recall risks once they are over. I
> remember a guy was saying he never had side effects and that he was fine
> and then we were talking about things and he said that that had done an
> HIV trial for a medication and he had jaundice because it stayed in his liver.
> He didn't think of it as a side effect, he probably didn't like to think about
> the whole instance. So, I think that it is pretty rare, pretty extreme, but I
> wonder how much of this tendency comes out. They want to make their
> money, they don't want to think about the humiliations and the risks they
> had been through, and maybe they end up being a little dishonest about the
> risk with themselves. So, taking that into account I am not sure about how
> to go about risks.—SHON, 2 JUNE 2004

There is no phase I clinical trial research without risk. The trial is designed as a controlled experiment that intends to produce basic knowledge related to the safety of the drug. Since the drug has until then only
been tested in animal species, questions remain about how the chemical
compound will behave in a human organism. The only way to answer
these questions entails a certain degree of risk for volunteers. In the past

trials were conducted on "captive" populations, specifically prison inmates. The more recent use of market-recruited, professional guinea pigs as research subjects raises questions concerning the way risk is understood and dealt with by this population.

In Shon's account, risk perception at first seems very straightforward and unproblematic. Experienced guinea pigs in general have not encountered major adverse effects while volunteering in the trials, and other occupations pursued by guinea pigs seem riskier. But then Shon admits that volunteers sometimes do not want to think about risks once the trial is over. He insinuates that the need to keep doing trials might lead volunteers to overlook the risks posed by trials. As a result of this realization, he seems much less certain about risk perception among volunteers and is unable to offer a definite statement. Shon's first approach to the risks of trials is shared by most volunteers, who focus on immediate risks without giving much thought to the long term, and his ambiguity about risk assessment is fairly uncommon among professional volunteers.

Shon made his remarks about long-term effects, or LTEs, almost at the end of my fieldwork, and they were the first evidence I had that veteran guinea pigs gave any thought to the subject. Until that moment I had often asked both anarchist and non-anarchist guinea pigs about LTEs, and always received the same answer: the drug in the blood washes away a few days after the trial is over and does not appear in either blood or urine tests. More inexperienced volunteers would add that they did not plan to depend on trials income forever: they had better ideas for their future.

It thus seemed as if the concerns I had about long-term effects were not shared by anyone else in the guinea pig community. But this was not true. In such a close-knit community I got to know some of my informants' female friends, and they confided to me that they had a great deal of concern about both the immediate and long-term effects of clinical trials. One friend told me that her partner was "catching every virus around because his immune system is weakened by the trials." She said that he was "always sick," that she had asked him many times to "leave the trials and get a regular eight-dollars job," but that he continued to do trials because of the income and because he thought the trials were "cool . . . alternative, contra-cultural stuff and all that."

The professionalization of phase I clinical subjects led to the formation of a steady market-recruited group employed regularly as human subjects. One of the most pressing issues connected to their participation was the relation between risks and these commoditization processes.

ANTHROPOLOGY OF RISK: RISK SOCIETY, "REFLEXIVE MODERNITY," AND GOVERNMENTALITY THEORIES OF RISK

In the last two decades the social sciences have seen risk studies emerge as a new area of disciplinary interest. Risk has been perceived as an essential part of "reflexive modernity" (Beck 1992; Beck, Giddens, and Lash 1994; Giddens 1990) in postindustrial societies. Central to Beck's and Giddens's writings on risk is the notion that late modernity is characterized by a critique of the processes of modernity, which are no longer unproblematically viewed as producing "goods" but are now seen to produce many of the dangers of "bads" from which we feel threatened. The central institutions of late modernity—government, industry, science—are singled out as the main producers of risks. An emphasis on risk, Beck and Giddens assert, is thus an integral feature of a society that has come to reflect upon and critique itself. An important point made by these authors is that institutions make decisions that place citizens at risk but are not accountable for doing so. Individuals do not seek to live in a world without risk, which according to Beck and Giddens is impossible, but to have a say in the type and levels of risk with which they may be forced to live.

A similar approach to risk is based on Foucault's writings on governmentality. This approach focuses not on investigating the nature of risk itself but rather on the forms of knowledge, the dominant discourses and expert techniques and institutions that serve to render risk calculable and knowledgeable, bringing it into being. Risk is a way—or rather, a set of different ways—of ordering reality, or rendering it into calculable form. It is a way of representing events so that they might be made governable in particular ways, with particular techniques and for particular goals (Dean 1999).

While these approaches offer valuable social and political clues to understanding how risk is constructed, they have been criticized for operating at the level of grand theory, with little use of empirical work on how people conceptualize and experience risks as part of their everyday lives (Lupton 1999). In spite of these critiques, the various approaches to risk offer valuable insights into how society manages the ethics and risks of using guinea pigs in clinical-trials research, and how accountability for risk is apportioned by such powerful institutions as the pharmaceutical industry and the Food and Drug Administration, whose risk assessments, technical but also political, might subject volunteers to risks beyond their control. And of course GPZ provides an example of the professional guinea pig's "reflexivity," offering their own understandings of the risks they face as paid subjects.

A significant event that contributed to a more empirical understanding of risk in the social sciences was the emergence of AIDS in the 1980s, forcing social scientists to identify and measure the risk of sexual practices and intravenous drug use. Some of the theorizations on risk presented here are heavily influenced by these efforts and draw their empirical support from AIDS data.

THE BEHAVIORAL APPROACH TO RISK

The behavioral approach to risk emerged in the 1980s, heavily influenced by behavioral social psychology. Two of the most widely used models are the health belief model (Becker and Joseph 1988) and the theory of reasoned action (Ajzen and Fishbein eds. 1980). Here individual behaviors are the only determinants of individual health. In turn, individual risk behaviors are explained by individuals' risk perceptions. According to the behavioral approach there is a direct relationship between beliefs and practices, so that if people have correct information about the risks and how to avoid them, they will rationally choose to change their behavior. Critics have argued that individual beliefs are not the only determinants of individual practices. Information in itself is insufficient to produce risk-reducing behavioral change. People take decisions and act in particular social contexts, and these contexts cannot be neglected as the behavioral theories would have us do (Parker, Barbosa, and Aggleton 2000). The social context shapes the way risks are perceived and also influences the ways we respond to them. Furthermore, the context imposes limits on the courses of action that any one individual can choose and implement (Singer 1994; Singer 1998; Clatts, Deren, and Friedman 1991).

Professional guinea pigs support Parker's view. They construct a risk hierarchy, with certain trials like those involving experimental psychiatric drugs at the top, and the testing of drugs already on the market, like painkillers, near the bottom. My research with paid guinea pigs shows that experienced volunteers who had participated in at least one trial that they knew presented an unusually high risk level had been enticed by the financial rewards. Thus they made their choice in a social context characterized by economic constraints: the need to maintain a certain lifestyle, or financial inducements, may have led these volunteers to discount accurate information about a particular drug trial.

All the remaining approaches to the study of risk have some similarities, continuities, and contradictions, but they all converge to support the idea that risks cannot be understood unless they are placed in a broader sociocultural context that surpasses the individual level postulated by the behavioral epidemiological approach.

THE CULTURAL APPROACH TO RISK

The cultural approach to risk is represented by authors like Mary Douglas who stress the cultural determinants of risks in opposition to the individual, cognitive, and utilitarian approaches emphasized by the behavioral epidemiological and rational choice models. Douglas argues that risk is not a natural, fixed category but instead has to be understood as culturally, socially, and historically constructed. Every society selects and reacts to a particular set of risks. She notes that the selection and reaction of a particular hazard shows essential features of the social organization of a society (Douglas 1992).

The cultural approach illustrates Douglas's concern for groups and institutions and their role in maintaining a particular form of social organization. Critics of the cultural approach to suggest that its emphasis on institutions instead of individuals misses a crucial point: not all individuals are equally exposed to risk. As the political economy approach to risk shows, it is usually the poor and disenfranchised who are placed disproportionately at risk (Baer, Singer, and Susser 2003; Singer and Baer 2009; Singer 2006; Farmer, Connors, and Simmons eds. 1996; Farmer 2002). This pattern is illustrated by the past use in biomedical research of human subjects taken from captive populations such as orphans, the mentally enfeebled, and prisoners, and the present use of poor, disenfranchised paid volunteers.

Another weakness in this approach is that it emphasizes normative aspects, neglecting, for example, strategic relations among members in the immediate social situation (Bellaby 1990). These points are central to the theorists of the situated rationality approach to risk. An important contribution from these theorists is the realization that social interactions among volunteers shape individual experiences and understandings of the trials and the ways risk is constructed and dealt with.

Despite these critiques the cultural approach to risk is very significant for the social sciences, because it goes beyond a view of risk that focuses on the individual and her or his psychological or cognitive responses to risk, and in doing so considers the sociocultural context in which individuals are situated and in which they make judgments about risk.

THE SITUATED RATIONALITY APPROACH

The situated rationality theory outlines the situational elements that individuals consider when adopting a particular behavior (Connors 1996). This approach emphasizes the immediate social and interactional elements present in the social context in which individuals act and take decisions about risks. It proposes that individuals are influenced by the immediate benefits related to risk behaviors. While this theory is inspired by the rational choice approach to risk, there are some important differences. Contrary to the rational choice actor, the individual here is not an abstract and detached one but instead someone influenced by the aesthetic, emotional, and interactional elements present in his or her social context. As this ethnography shows, a volunteer's decision about entering a trial is based overwhelmingly on financial considerations. Volunteers calculate the hourly, daily, and total income potentially derived from a trial. They also consider the convenience of the location, the duration of the trial, and the risk level. But unlike the rational choice subject, the volunteer weighs these criteria in close interaction with other volunteers. As previously noted, risk assessment is not an individual but a social process. Familiarity with trial sites and the need to enroll with friends or acquaintances volunteering for the same trial are also persuasive facts.

The situated rationality approach is much more interested in explaining its own data than in elaborating a more general theory of risk practices. The emphasis on the immediate benefits of risk behavior, such as financial reward, is also perceived to be an obstacle for a broader application.

THE POLITICAL ECONOMY APPROACH TO RISK

The political economy approach to risk emphasizes social, structural, and historical processes reinforcing social inequalities as the main elements for understanding how individuals perceive and deal with risk. Authors like Singer, Clatts, and Susser discard the cognitive and individual epidemiological approach to risk, stressing how "risky social behavior is shaped by external social and economic context" (Singer 1998). Clatts's study of HIV risk perceptions among intravenous drug users in Harlem shows that factors such as poverty and social marginalization are linked to how individuals perceive and deal with the risks. Any intervention program, Clatts suggests, should take into consideration the behavioral shift that individuals must effect, and the underlying social inequalities, or else it will have a poor chance of success.

The authors who propose a political economy approach to risk have extended their inquiry into health risks in industrial settings (Susser 1988; Singer and Baer 2008). Experiences like those at Love Canal and Three Mile Island in the United States, Bhopal in India, and Chernobyl in Ukraine (Petryna 2002) have increased awareness of the risks that industry poses to workers and residents in areas surrounding factories. The political economy approach to industrial risk argues that the industry has historically disregarded workers' health, both when state regulation was absent in earlier years and when it was present in later years. According to Susser, the level and kind of occupational health risks to which workers are exposed is related to the historical development of industry, shifts in worker and management relationships, and state regulation. In addition, social movements beyond the workplace influence working conditions and the existence of industrial hazards and should also be considered in assessing industrial risk.

As previously noted, the political economy approach argues that social inequalities expose certain people to disproportionate risk. To earn a livelihood, the poor and disenfranchised face risks that they may not recognize or are unwilling to forgo. Professional guinea pigs are just one example. Their dependence on the income, mobility, and lack of shared experiences at the same workplace over a long period makes them less aware of long-term risk than coal miners and asbestos workers.

The goal of any risk analysis should be to account for the material, economic, historical, and social constraints facing each decision-making agent, without leaving behind the symbolic dimensions of that agent's experiences of risks and the ways they can provide agents with the power to contest or control their situation more efficiently.

In sum, the behavioral epidemiological model on risk, which at its core is individualistic, cognitive, and utilitarian, neglects the social contexts in which individuals live and make decisions about risks. The other perspectives discussed above offer different contributions to the study of risk in clinical-trials research, but no single approach can account for the multidimensional way in which risks are perceived and dealt with by the industry and human volunteers. I stress the need to go beyond the notion of a universal "risk subject" that tends to appear, particularly in the risk society and governmentality perspectives. Responses to risk may be understood as aesthetic, affective, and hermeneutic phenomena, grounded in everyday experiences and social relationships (Lash 1993). I believe that a better understanding is needed of how risk logics are produced and operate at the level of situated experience. We need to know more about how the structuring factors of gender, ethnicity, age, and social class, as well as different social contexts such as the different phases and experiences of trials, influence risk logics.

While all but the behavioral perspectives emphasize the social, cultural, and political nature of risk, they offer somewhat differently nuanced approaches to the phenomenon of risk as a socially constructed phenomenon. Indeed they may be placed along a continuum, with technical and scientific approaches at one pole and a highly relativist constructionist approach at the other. Whether risks are to be understood as constructed or objective realities is important. My position is that risks are socially constructed but are also a significant presence in the lives of any subjects volunteering for any trial. The painful and unnecessary deaths of human subjects in the last several years is a sad remainder that risks are not merely social constructions and that volunteers risk their well-being when they decide to join the trial economy.

RISK PERCEPTION AMONG PROFESSIONAL GUINEA PIGS

As Mary Douglas reminds us, risks are individually perceived but socially constructed. Risk in the context of clinical trials research is understood by disciplines such as medicine, epidemiology, and pharmacology as a quantitative, bounded, and discrete phenomenon that can be objectively measured and dealt with. According to this techno-scientific perspective risks can be expressed statistically, providing the basis for neutral decisions about causation, safety, and dosage. However, social scientists have shown that assessing risk in clinical-trials research is a contingent social process.

Focusing on the way scientists detect adverse drug reactions at the trials and in post-marketing phases, Corrigan argues that scientific knowledge and practices are shaped by epistemological, political, and institutional arrangements to produce the scientists' risk assessments. Although scientists present their findings as "ready-made," that is, finished and stable, risk assessments are fluid and dependent upon a kind of knowledge that is always in the making. Abraham argues that adverse drug reactions are not neutrally assessed, as scientists claim; in fact the scientific assessment of some drug trials has been influenced by pharmaceutical companies' financial interests, which contribute to the process of ignoring, dismissing, or obfuscating unfavorable results.

Human subjects' understanding of risk in phase I research has not been studied. However, there are some studies of volunteers in later phases of drug development. These studies are centered in particular on the informed-consent process and examine such questions as how lay and professional perceptions of risk differ, the role that conflicts of interests play in the way risks are communicated to the volunteers, and the influence of biographical and illness trajectories in patients' decisions about risk taking.

Risk perception among professional guinea pigs is shaped by their clinical trial experiences and interactions with other volunteers. In this sense risk perception is closely related to the socialization of the professional guinea pig. Paid subjects share narratives of which trials represent risk and which do not, and of how to deal with risk. Local knowledge shapes the social construction of risk and the strategies that volunteers choose for coping with the risks they perceive.

A quick reference to guinea pigs' jokes about risk provides clues into the socially constructed character of risk in this population. Humorous tales describing bizarre experiments, or risky situations, form part of the guinea pig folklore. For example, some jokes depict an operation to remove and reinstall the pinky toe for $5,000, or to remove the heart and "put it back" for $10,000. These jokes, according to *Guinea Pig Zero*, were first circulated by the head researcher at Jefferson and quickly picked up by professional guinea pigs. The popularity of the jokes reflects paid subjects' awareness of how their own bodies were commodified and their anxieties about the risks they might face as paid subjects.

Volunteers not only share jokes about risk but more importantly information about risk. It is not unusual for volunteers in the West Philly community to consult each other about the potential risks of a prospective trial, especially if the drug has not yet been tested in humans. Volunteers may also search the Internet or consult people with medical training if they have doubts about a drug being tested.

The process of signing the informed-consent form at the beginning of a trial provides the best opportunity for those administering the trial to disclose risks to volunteers. This document details the design, procedures, risks, and benefits of the study and is perceived by volunteers to be the main source of information about the trial. Close interaction among volunteers is facilitated by the informed-consent process, the screening, and especially the lengthy inpatient trials, which provide less experienced members an opportunity to expand their understanding of the way trials are organized, which risks they might face, and how to deal with risk.

The social construction of risk among professional guinea pigs is constructed along two dimensions: a temporal dimension along which risks range from short-term to long-term, and a severity dimension, along which risks range from low to high. Paid subjects' concerns are located in the present and are related only to the trial for which they are currently volunteering and its short-term effects. Helms elaborates: "Nobody thinks a lot about long-term risks. It is like getting a job in a restaurant, the neighborhood with a lot of crime, a faraway train, whatever. You are thinking about a short-term problem, you are not thinking about what is going to bother you five years from now. You are thinking how am I gonna get to this job and now I am getting my weekly paycheck for this job. And with a trial is the same thing. You are not thinking that these things are going to give you cancer five years from now, or that you might have a high level of radiation in your body" (Helms, 5 January 2005). As Helms observes, volunteers are not thinking that they might become ill years after the trial. Instead, they are worried about short-term considerations such as acceptance into the trial, and then focusing on the schedule and their financial compensation.

As for the severity of risk, paid subjects perceive most clinical trials as presenting a moderate risk. They see the trials as carefully controlled, with risk levels further limited by the ethical regulations governing the use of human subjects. In their experience, serious adverse effects and dangerous situations are exceptional. A subject wanting to join a particularly low-risk study would look for one involving a drug already on the market that presented few or no side effects, even at the high doses administered during a trial—perhaps a pain reliever similar to Tylenol. Yet even professional guinea pigs are aware that there are uncertainties associated with any experimental trial, and that scientists do not know everything about any drug, its risks, and its side effects. Thus in my survey of risk perception, when asked about the risk levels of trials, volunteers tended to assess risk levels as moderate instead of low. Non-volunteers and the general public, familiar with past and present abuses in biomedical and clinical-trials research, perceive trials as being more risky than they are.

While the majority of the trials are placed in the medium risk category by volunteers, some trials are perceived as presenting a high risk. Volunteers perceive experimental drugs as riskier than marketed drugs. They are reassured that a drug on the market has already been tested in several trials and later by an even larger population after reaching the market. In contrast, experimental drugs do not offer this safeguard, according to trial subjects. New experimental drugs, in particular those that change the immunological system, and psychiatric drugs that alter the chemical structure of the brain, are considered high-risk. "I definitely prefer to do drug studies with drugs that are already in the market and sometimes I took experimental drugs. But again, there is that thing where a marketed HIV or psych drug might have a lot more risk than an investigational drug that is only a blood thinner. What I would ask when I was in a study is: what would this drug do to me chemically? If it thins or straightens my blood I am not that worried about it. But if it does affect my mind or significantly affects the chemistry of my body, that's more of a risk than a blood thinner or a bone strengthener" (Spam, 28 July 2004). Experimental studies involving genetic drug testing and sleep deprivation are also a source of major concern. While some volunteers' views that experimental drugs present a higher risk is shared by scientists, the way volunteers understand and deal with risk is heavily influenced by local knowledge about their bodies and biological processes.

Guinea Pig Zero published a series of horror stories about volunteers' experiences in trials for experimental drugs, especially psychiatric drugs. "A drug has to stay in your body to interact with another drug but it washes out in a few days. It is gone so it is not going to interact with something that you are going to take later. Think of this, if you smoke half a pack of cigarettes a day and a couple of beers a day you are way ahead, miles and miles ahead of me than doing a guinea pig study on carefully controlled situations, very clear dosages. If it is one of these high-risk studies like studying a new kind of Paxil, Prozac or something, then you are really in the Wild West. You are taking a ridiculous risk and it is too bad that some people go for it—a lot of people are—it is even worse that people are sponsoring studies and try to make money on garbage that is dangerous and it doesn't help anybody" (Helms, 15 January 2004). Here, as Helms suggests, volunteers enter uncharted territory. He elaborates on why psychiatric drug trials are to be avoided:

> Psychiatric trials are for a couple of reasons very different from trials of non-psychotropic drugs because they involve your mind. You are renting your mind and your body at the same time instead of just your body. It is a completely different economic deal. Secondly, in the psychotropic drug trials, people are writing diseases into existence. You cannot fake fast heartbeat into existence; you cannot make people believe that the heart is beating faster. I put a stethoscope into your chest and check your fucking heartbeat, that's simple. They cannot invent your blood pressure but they can invent your depression, they can invent your mood. And they can change the interpretation of what you say according to what the drug market wants. The marketing department writes the label of the drug, not the fucking doctors, the scientists. It is the marketing department. And they also write the disclaimers, fight the lawsuits. Blame the disease, not the drug. Like, he is getting into middle age, a lot of time on his hands and is getting a little raunchy goes into the psychiatrist for a little talk, gets put on Prozac and two weeks later he slaughters the whole family with a rifle and blows his own brain out. Tell me it is not the fucking Prozac! That is what I think, fuck you, fuck you. And it happens over and over again and the lawsuits get buried by companies that put a lot of money to quiet people down.

Helms's strong opinion about psychiatric drugs echoes the concerns of other professional guinea pigs and contrasts with the usual, more neutral, way they talk about risks. The wariness of the anarchist community toward psychiatric drugs reflects its hostility toward the industry, which it sees as "writing diseases into existence," at considerable risk to both volunteers and patients, in a search for profits. For the anarchist guinea pig community of West Philadelphia, trials of psychiatric drugs also have more direct and personal connotations. One disturbing event occurred in December 1995 when a former professional guinea pig, an experienced volunteer and well-known local activist, enrolled in a trial for the antidepressant Paxil and the antihistamine Seldane, with tragic results. This event had such a profound impact on the community that Helms issued a report card for the research site where the trial took place, bearing the headline: "Brain-sluts, look no further: GSK Corporate Control in All of its Glory." The report card assigned a "dirty" D to the facility, noting that while the pay was good and the trials generally of short duration, "the catch is that your mental health is not very important to these researchers." The trial subject, according to the account, "emerged with $7,000 in his pocket but his mind in Planet Zork," having experienced a "life-changing mental breakdown." According to Helms, the facility enrolled the volunteer in a new experimental trial in June of the following year, just a few months after the first trial ended.

The volunteer's fellow professional guinea pigs remember him as being "delusional," hallucinating, paranoid, and clearly losing touch with reality. For example, he insisted that the movie *Twelve Monkeys* conveyed a militant message to the radical community of anarchists in West Philly to organize to overthrow the United States government using bacteriological and chemical weapons. Nobody took his suggestion seriously. In another episode, the volunteer tried to buy a dilapidated house to start a new community, but he falsified transaction documents and in the end his friends had to bail him out with money from their own pockets. These events, along with his mood swings, anxieties, and antisocial behavior, ended up alienating him from his best friends, forcing him to abandon the West Philly anarchist community. Some former friends believe that he is in Italy; others think he might be in Australia. The story was relevant enough to the West Philly anarchist community for it to be published in GPZ. Anarchist guinea pigs who knew the volunteer personally all mentioned the case to me. Even some volunteers who came later to the area referred to the case to make a point about the danger of psychiatric-drug trials.

The persistent social memory of this single event many years later suggests that the story has some iconic value. I suggest that the narrative operates as a cautionary tale among anarchist professional guinea pigs about the abuses of the pharmaceutical industry and the risks of volunteering for trials that "mess up your mind."

RISK AND THE PROFESSIONALIZATION OF THE GUINEA PIG SUBJECT

The volunteers' identities are shaped by their definition of guinea pigging as work. This is especially true of the anarchist community of West Philadelphia, although it applies to some other self-defined professional guinea pigs as well. The commodification of clinical trials research has formed a group of reliable, knowledgeable, and willing subjects who depend on participation in trials for income to support themselves. Rajan describes a similar process among unemployed textile workers in Mumbai who work as experimental subjects for genetic trials. He argues that as experimental subjects they enter into systems of capital as a source of value creation and as a source of scientific knowledge production (Rajan 2005).

But to become a professional research subject in this double sense, subjected to capital as well as to science, the volunteer must remain for some time in the trial economy. One-time participation does not constitute professional guinea pigging. As shown earlier, the disciplined body is an indispensable requirement of the professional research subject, and it is for this reason that professional participants are being sought and rewarded by the industry. But there is another element that plays a central role in the transition from volunteer to professional guinea pig: subjects need to perceive the risks they face as not too high, or otherwise they might not continue in the trial economy.

Volunteers with just a few trials seem to show some concern about the risk faced in trials and also mention possible long-term effects (LTE). Routinization, however, leads to diminished concern on both counts. Dependency on trial income, trial experiences that have not exposed them to side effects, and interactions with more experienced volunteers convinces newcomers that risks are not to be feared. Also, as volunteers move along in their careers as guinea pigs they gain experiences that contribute not only to their risk perception but also to a shared narrative about risks. "I don't think I did many studies that might have LTE. I didn't do studies that had a pretty bad LTE in my body chemistry. So, I am not that worried about it. No. Also, it's hard to tell too but there is so much fucking toxic stuff around, at work, I lived around oil refineries, I lived in an old house, I used to work with this chemical, I used to work with that chemical. I don't know if an LTE shows up I would be able to tell where it came from. No, I am not that worried" (Spam, 28 July 2004).

Such perceptions influence guinea pigs' practices, and practices shape their perceptions. The notion that some trials are risky might dissuade volunteers from joining. And continual participation in trials can produce changes in perceptions.

Thus as they become more engaged and dependent on the trial economy, volunteers' understandings of the trial and its risks change. Beginners are more worried about risks than professionals. Maybe this reflects the general population's anxieties about biomedical research and its well-publicized abuses. Volunteers' initial uneasiness focuses on the unknown effects of the drugs, but it also reflects a discomfort with a procedure they do not yet fully understand. In addition, volunteers are concerned about potential long-term risks. Some volunteers mentioned that they were somewhat concerned about developing cancer in the future.

As less experienced volunteers become socialized into the role of the professional guinea pig and interact with more experienced workers, and as their own experience involves no serious adverse drug reactions (ADRs), they adopt the common professional narrative about how to understand and handle risk. Their risk sensibilities become more focused on particular trials, such as trials involving psychiatric medication, genetic drugs, and sleep deprivation. At the same time, routinization leads them to minimize or deny long-term risks.

As we have seen, anarchist volunteers tend to compare their risks with those they have faced or would face in industrial or service jobs, or in industrial accidents involving chemicals or heavy machinery. They also consider the risks that the general public shoulders when taking drugs. This evaluation reflects their ethical views rather than those of the pharmaceutical industry. According to professional guinea pigs, patients taking marketed drugs are "unaware" and are in fact unpaid guinea pigs, since the drugs they take may have adverse side effects not detected in experimental trials with small samples. Vioxx and many other drugs that have been retired from the market because of unacceptable risks for patients give some credence to this belief.

RISK MANAGEMENT STRATEGIES AMONG PROFESSIONAL GUINEA PIGS

Professional guinea pigs believe that risk can be known and managed. This perspective is based on their trial experiences and understandings; it helps volunteers to sustain their confidence, but it can also keep them volunteering. Local knowledge influences the way risk is constructed and how volunteers manage risk.

The local classification of risk hierarchies is one way volunteers attempt to manage anxiety. They avoid trials at the top of their risk hierarchy, even quitting the trial if unforeseen risks arise. If a trial is perceived as being very high-risk, volunteers may avoid the trial altogether. Experienced volunteers say they have at least once turned down a trial because they felt that it presented unacceptable risks. Even so, most experienced guinea pigs have done at least one trial that they perceived as "too risky," enticed by the promise of substantial financial gain.

For the anarchist professional guinea pig community some of these concerns are less acute than for paid subjects from elsewhere. Volunteers from outside the city must pay travel and housing expenses—usually in cheap places like the youth hostel where I met KingLabRat and the Canadian Guinea Pig—along with living costs while they wait to find out if they will be accepted into the trial. Once they are accepted the inpatient trial regimen covers most of their material needs, but it also influences their ability to decide whether to stay in the trial if something goes unexpectedly. Until you get a check, the pharmaceutical companies sponsoring the trials "have you by the balls," as the Canadian Guinea Pig told me. By contrast, the anarchist guinea pigs are single, with no children, have their own living arrangements, and face less pressure to undertake risks or trial conditions they feel are not acceptable.

A more extreme version of risk management is to abandon the trial. This is a very rare measure, and professional guinea pigs use it as a last resort. Sometimes a drug has secondary effects that are harder than the volunteers expected. If a volunteer manages to show that these effects are the direct result of the trial, then he or she may be able to leave, sometimes receiving full payment, or a pro-rated portion. While there is no penalty attached to leaving a trial in such circumstances, making the case is not easy, and failure to do so can be financially costly for participants.

Some professional guinea pigs believe that certain substances help them to "clean the blood" and "detoxify" the body of the chemicals absorbed during a trial. They assume that the chemical substances are only contained in the blood and urine. If a few days after the drug intake is finished the drug remains cannot be found in tests, then volunteers assume that none remains in their bodies. This assumption is shared by most professional guinea pigs, which helps to explain why they do not give a lot of attention to their "cleansing" practices other than drinking water, a standard procedure usually suggested by the nurses or doctors conducting the trials. Volunteers do resort to other cleansing methods on special occasions, for example after a very long and demanding trial when they fear that the drug administered had a particular toxicity, or if they are planning to do another trial soon after finishing the first. Cleansing practices are also based on local knowledge about volunteers' bodies and their interactions with the substances ingested during the trials.

Scott, an experienced volunteer living in the anarchist community, explains some of his methods: "There are a couple of times where I didn't wait what I was supposed to wait. Like I did one two weeks after the other or something. I make sure to drink a lot of water and actually took some herbs in those cases. One of the best ways to clean up your system is lots of water, of course, and then goldenseal and then non-sugar cranberry juice. The combination of that stuff would wash you out. So, I did that and I thought that I was reasonably safe doing that. I don't remember what the drugs were but they didn't seem risky" (Scott, 3 June 2004). Unsweetened cranberry juice is a standard drink for professional guinea pigs and is believed to help absorb, metabolize, and eliminate toxic trial substances. In addition, herbs like goldenseal and marigold flowers were suggested by GPZ as ways of "keeping the blood fresh and clean." Goldenseal, according to the zine, is "said to have a dramatic cleansing power, and is recommended by herbalists for removing the toxins related to alcohol, coffee, nicotine and other substances from blood."

A small group of volunteers in the anarchist community sometimes attempt diets that involve eating only apples for several days, or yogurt, in the belief that this also helps "clean" their bodies. The use of herbs and organic methods of cleansing is preferred in the anarchist community. Although anarchist volunteers usually eat meat in the trials, mainly because they are required to do so, they place a high value on vegetables, organic diets, and healing practices. Professional subjects not affiliated with the anarchist group prefer a chemical approach, using blood supplements that contain iron, which helps rebuild the blood supply. KingLab-Rat is almost a walking infomercial for iron supplements, which he uses extensively to cleanse his blood so as to be able to volunteer for another trial as soon as possible:

> If you volunteer in another trial before time they might find out, they might know but sometimes you can pull it off. When they do the blood work, urine work, they'll know because if your system is not properly flushed it will be in your system. So you have to wait seven to ten days to have your drug flushed out. If you are physically fit and you take care of your blood work you could jump into another study seven to ten days after you finish one. We have stuff on the market that works, replenishes your blood, iron supplements. I take it specially when I come out of a long trial where I had a lot of blood drawn. This thing really guarantees to build up your red blood cells. Everything in your body is being taken care of by fluids. The fluids are the only thing that gets into every micro-cell of your body. This Elixir takes care of anything at the micro-cell level in your body, even into your bones. So take that, put it into a shot glass before a meal and it'll do the trick. You will feel it working. A lot of people is taking this, they dropped the pills and got the bottle. I am satisfied with myself because I accomplished what many people cannot get: I managed to live comfortably. (KingLabRat, 16 February 2004)

Despite their attempts to manage risk, professional guinea pigs are placed at considerable harm when they remain in trials for many years, exposing themselves to potentially synergistic drug interactions and long-term effects. The social organization of the clinical trials and the guinea pigs' lifestyle make it more difficult for them to become aware of these interactions and of effects that may appear many years after a trial is completed. While volunteers maintain close interaction during the trials, which might last from a few days up to a few weeks, once a trial is over volunteers usually do not remain in contact. Some leave for other cities looking for new trial opportunities. Even the more stable community of professional anarchist guinea pigs in Philadelphia is highly mobile and in constant flux. This fact contrasts with the stability of other categories of workers performing toxic or dangerous trades such as coal miners, or those exposed to asbestos or other industrial pollutants. It was only over extended periods of sharing experiences that these workers developed an awareness of risk, in contrast to the reassurances offered by the industry. But for professional guinea pigs, their mobility and relative anonymity conspire against this possibility. Their situation resembles that of migrant agricultural workers who face similar risks associated with agro-toxics. The lack of a centralized register of human subjects in phase I trials might also obscure the existence of the problem for the pharmaceutical industry and regulatory agencies like the FDA. In addition, the pharmaceutical industry has no incentive to invest in research to study long-term effects and synergistic risks.

4

BIG PHARMA AND HIV CLINICAL TRIALS

A Case Study

COMMUNITY-BASED TRIAL ORGANIZATION (CBTO)

CBTO occupies a five-story terracotta building in downtown Philadelphia. The street, filled with nicely kept colonial houses, is close to the historic district and like the surrounding neighborhood has undergone intensive gentrification since the mid-1990s. Still, its central location is perfect to serve its "customers," mostly poor, African American HIV patients. This institution is a large community-based center for AIDS research, also providing health care for poor HIV patients, education, and advocacy.

As the HIV epidemic grew it generated a powerful social response that led community members to organize to fight against the disease, inspired by the conviction that progress against AIDS could not be made if efforts to develop effective drugs and vaccines were left to the pharmaceutical industry alone. CBTO and the larger national network to which it belonged would engage in trials that the industry was perceived as uninterested in pursuing because of their lack of immediate profitability. In addition, Act-Up, a social movement intended to support the cause of AIDS, established an informal but close relationship with CBTO when one of its members joined CBTO's educational section. CBTO can be seen as the result of neoliberal management of the epidemic, in particular the practice of states and cities of transferring to community organizations the responsibility for fighting the epidemic and the resources needed to do so.

The physical changes at its facilities offer a glimpse into the transformation of CBTO from community research site managed by activists and occupying a small room at the Graduate Hospital in the late 1980s to its current role in providing health care, HIV research, and advocacy. As its function has changed, CBTO has had to balance activism with the rhetoric and practices of a service organization devoted to the consumers' well-being.

CBTO started as part of the Community Research Initiative, which in 1987 obtained a grant from the American Fund to support community-based AIDS research. The grant was requested by a gay endocrinologist treating AIDS patients in the belief that without community involvement, therapeutic advances in drug research would be much harder to achieve. CBTO joined the Community Research Initiative effort in 1990, occupying a small office space at the Graduate Hospital of the University of Pennsylvania in downtown Philadelphia.

For the first four years CBTO did only community-based research as part of the Community Research Initiative network, but in 1995 a grant from Community Programs for Clinical Research on AIDS (CPCRA) allowed it to expand its community-based research. Its staff grew from four to ten, including its director, one administrative position, and seven members of the research team. The grant also allowed CBTO to move to half of the fifth floor at its current location and it provided funds to hire a community activist for an education and advocacy program for patients living with HIV.

In 1996 CBTO's board president died, bequeathing funds which allowed for the opening of a treatment center in the following year, filling the space contiguous to the research area. In 2000 a grant from the Robert Wood Johnson Foundation made it possible for CBTO to hire its principal investigator (PI) as its full-time medical director. Around the same time the research lab that was crowding the fifth floor along with the treatment center moved to a new space in the first floor.

While during its first years the CBTO board was composed of doctors, currently there are no doctors on the board. According to CBTO's director and a board member, the composition of the board reflects the institution's role as a minority provider. Most board members are African American descent and from one-third to half are living with HIV. The director of CBTO summarizes the board's composition: "Lots of different people. We just don't have a lot of rich people."

Clinical trials are conducted at CBTO's research department. The lobby accommodates a copy machine, a couple of seats, and a desk sometimes occupied by a secretary. Pens displaying the logos of HIV drugs are used by patients to fill out a sign-in sheet. One wall has a Viracept clock and close to it a poster announces the SMART study, with information about "Joining a Global AIDS Effort." Patients wait in the lobby until it is time for their appointment. Usually there are no more than a few patients visiting the facility every day. Sometimes there are one or two patients in the waiting room, but typically patients come to their scheduled appointments on time and do not have to wait. They ring a bell on an interior door and usually the head nurse or the phlebotomist comes to the door and lets them in. After walking through a room filled with cabinets and CPCRA files, used only occasionally for NIH and industry monitors, patients are ushered to a room to be interviewed and usually to have their blood taken. Although the research department houses three exam rooms, staff regularly uses only the one that has a cardiac monitor. In addition to a stretcher, all exam rooms have cabinets filled with needles, cotton, and supplies. The lab has a centrifuge to separate blood components, which are usually sent out for processing. The research space also uses two rooms as office space.

Staff members greet their patients by name and can identify which trial they are in. The stability of the staff and its continuous interaction with patients over periods as long as forty-eight to ninety-six weeks also builds personal relationships. Currently there are 128 patients in HIV trials research.

There are two types of trials being conducted at CBTO: community trials and industry trials. As a community-based research site, CBTO is part of the CPCRA network, which administers among other trials the Strategies for the Management of Anti-Retroviral Therapy (SMART) trial. The institution also serves as a research site for other community trials such as Wistar, conducted by the University of Pennsylvania. CBTO also conducts industry trials to test new drug regimens being developed by the pharmaceutical industry.

The PI oversees the care of the patients that come to the center and is in charge of almost all the industry trials that are currently active. An infectious disease doctor before coming to CBTO in 2001, he was a junior attending physician at Cooper Hospital in Philadelphia. During his experience at Cooper he was a co-investigator for HIV trials. The majority of the industry trials at CBTO are in phases III or IV, testing drugs already approved by the FDA or on the verge of being approved and placed in expanded access programs. While the PI notes that experimental drug trials are "of concern" because the researchers "don't have a clear idea about how are they going to interact with the host," he acknowledges that the main reason why these studies are not conducted at CBTO is lack of infrastructure. In particular, some of the studies require that patients stay overnight, and the facilities to do not allow for this.

Since 2000 twelve industry trials have been conducted at CBTO; currently five or six are scheduled. The PI summarizes the reasons for this growth: "There are more opportunities and our comfort level has increased, the comfort levels of our staffing during these trials has increased as well. There are more combinations of drugs being tested out there and the level of competition among pharmaceutical companies is big." The emergence of protease inhibitor drugs in the mid-1990s opened significant opportunities for drug development as well as for therapeutic interventions. While in the mid-1990s there were only a couple of protease inhibitor drugs, currently there are more than twenty AIDS drugs available and many more in the pipeline. More drugs also mean more possibilities of drug combinations, which also must be tested. According to the PI there is an additional reason for the emergence of HIV drug trials: "Everyone wants to show that their drug is the preferred one, so there is a lot of competition, so there are more trials."

One of the most important trials being performed as part of the CPCRA network is the SMART trial, being coordinated by the head nurse of the research department. It is a six- to nine-year study intended to assess whether HIV patients can interrupt their treatments over extended periods without compromising their health. CBTO is part of an international network of research sites in North America, Europe, Asia, and South America that enrolls more than fifteen hundred volunteers. The study attempts to enroll nearly six thousand in the coming years. (A few months after I finished my fieldwork the SMART trial was discontinued ahead of schedule—it was supposed to end in 2006—after findings indicated that the temporary interruption of antiretroviral therapy presented high risks for volunteers.)

The head nurse joined CBTO as a clinical research coordinator in May 2001. Before this she had worked at the HIV unit of the University of Pennsylvania's Graduate Hospital since 1992. In addition to taking care of the patients, she also engaged in clinical trials at the facility, testing protease inhibitors among other drugs. Her interest in trial research increased after the completion of her master's degree. Joining CBTO's research department offered her an opportunity to further her research interests while still being able to work with HIV patients in an environment she described as "family." She is the project coordinator for the SMART study, responsible for supervision, quality assurance, budget preparation, liaison between the CBTO office and the network headquarters in Washington, and organizing meetings and conference calls.

INSTITUTIONAL REVIEW BOARD

Before a trial can be conducted at CBTO it must be reviewed by its IRB. Until 1997 research protocols had been sent out for review to big university hospitals in the city, which sometimes resulted in considerable delays, costing patients important research opportunities. To solve this problem, and to keep pace with the demands of growing research activities, CBTO decided to form its own in-house IRB, led by a lawyer from a community-based organization that provides legal advice and services to AIDS patients. The board currently has six additional members: three community representatives and three medical doctors from local university hospitals.

When the IRB reviews a protocol it focuses on the goals and design of the study, in particular the risks and benefits for the volunteers. It also makes sure that the informed-consent form adequately conveys essential information to the volunteers in lay, nontechnical language. Chapter 7 explores the role of CBTO's IRB as part of the informed-consent process, along with its views on commodification in HIV trials research. When an industry trial is proposed, the protocol must also be submitted to the central IRB of the company that promotes the trial. Each trial has its own data safety monitoring board (DSMB) that reviews the data being collected and is in charge of raising any problems that may arise in connection with the trial. Every adverse event is reported by the DSMB to the IRB of CBTO. "There is no way in which you can anticipate and predict a bad outcome but it is very important to have a system in place that is efficient and that could eventually monitor the progress of the trial and that's what the Data Safety Monitoring Board is meant for. To be able to monitor the safety closely of these patients and make sure that if there is any pattern, out there, that looks suspicious, this Data Safety Monitoring Board is able to unveil this pattern and try to address the issues and if they believe that the risks outnumber the benefits then they should stop the trial. That's what they do usually. It all depends on how vigilant we are, how good the system that we have in place is able to determine these risky patterns and unveil them" (PI, 27 April 2004). Industry trials conducted at CBTO are also monitored by the pharmaceutical industry. Monitors visit periodically, usually for twelve weeks to scrutinize the research and make sure there are no inconsistencies in the data.

According to the principal investigator of CBTO, no significant problems had been reported by industry monitors with trials being conducted at CBTO, except that some patients' records were not showing in the charts. "But you know, we haven't had any major problems. The only problem we have is patients fell through the cracks and not showing to the charts but we have not had any major adverse event."

RECRUITMENT

Volunteers for trials at CBTO are recruited in a number of ways. Most are patients at the CBTO health care center, and there are also volunteers from Presbyterian Hospital at the University of Pennsylvania. Others are referred by infectious disease doctors like Dr. Watkins, across the street from CBTO, who have patients that meet the criteria for trials. Doctors refer patients if they believe that they can benefit from a particular study. While most of the patients live in Philadelphia, the institution has been able to attract patients from New Jersey, Pennsylvania, and Florida. Volunteers reflect the demographics of the population served by CBTO: a majority of poor African American men and women, with some Latino and white volunteers. This composition is atypical of the nation as a whole, where HIV clinical-trials research has been conducted mostly on white males. The PI notes:

> It's important to study drugs and regimens in these patients because [they] respond to these drugs differently. So a regime that would be preferred in a Caucasian male might not be the best regime for an

African American male. And there is also the gender issue; we know that for certain drugs females tend to have more side effects than males; so also gender plays a role. Usually if you look at studies comparing regimes among themselves you have 70 to 80 percent males, 15 to 20 percent female. And usually you have 65 to 70 percent Caucasian and the rest are African Americans, Hispanics, and other minority groups. At CBTO we have 70 percent men and 30 percent women. That's good, we are reporting high on both.

We are very appealing because we have more minorities willing to enroll. And again, there is an element of financial gain in patients doing clinical trials, and unfortunately African Americans and Hispanics are poorer than the Caucasian population in general.

As in phase I trials, there is a need to recruit subjects for trials in the later phases of drug development. Sites with a potentially large body of volunteers are, as the PI recognizes, very appealing for the pharmaceutical industry, which needs to find thousands of patients to complete its drug trials. Usually large university research hospitals have both access to a large number of volunteers and the scientific expertise to conduct the trials. Smaller, specialized sites such as CBTO might also enter the network of HIV clinical-trials research for particular drug niches:

Well, the pharmaceutical companies decide who they want to choose in terms of sites, the way they wanted. Sometimes in considering the type of populations and also in terms of how they rate the site according to past experience, the credibility of the site, and the reputation of the site. So, they might come to us with a first-class study or a third-class study. Clearly the importance of these trials is ranked differently and the sites that are picked up to do these trials are ranked differently as well. A first-rate study picks first-rate sites to do it. We have been approached by all kinds of studies. I would rate them as first-rate, second-rate, and even sometimes third-rate studies and you know, it's up to us to decide if we are going to do the study or not but it's not up to us to decide if we are going to be picked up. Really, each study differs from the other and the pharmaceutical companies pick their sites based on who they believe it's gonna deliver and who's not gonna deliver. And if they have a study that it is too little, they want to pick up small sites that they think they can deliver. I tell you, if I had to rate my site I think that it's very competitive because we have the experience, we see a lot of patients in terms of HIV—obviously—and we have a record and a history of research. So they would want to work with us and that leads to novel therapies and novel strategies. (PI, 27 April 2004)

CBTO receives financial compensation for its enrollment in industry trials. According to the PI, the money paid to research sites is intended to compensate for direct costs like lab tests, as well as the time that researchers spend with paperwork, follow-up calls, and patients' visits.

There are two major categories, if you want, the researcher, the time that you are expending, the time that your staff is spending dealing with the situation and you have also costs of the bloodwork that you are doing. We take blood and many times instead of sending it to the central lab where the pharmaceutical company wants us to send it to, we do it in our lab instead. And this is costly and sometimes we need to do an X-ray too. Then there are direct and indirect costs. And then there is the effort of the researcher, researchers, in a sense. Our effort is based on the phone calls, the physicals that we do with the patient, encounters that we have with these patients.

The data belong to the industry that is doing the trial, so all that we do is provide them with the data and they analyze the data. So, we are compensated by the work that we are doing but I don't necessarily see this as a lucrative thing for us because if we think about it, I think that it is money-losing. (PI, 27 April 2004)

CBTO's PI and I developed a close relationship over time, and he was grateful to be able to present his point of view on the controversial issue of conflict of interest when a doctor doubles as a researcher. He revealed details of CBTO's operational budget to show that it made no profit and probably lost money doing industry trials. CBTO gets around $5,000 per patient enrolled in a trial, which might last from forty-eight to ninety-six weeks. All told, the share of CBTO's total revenue accounted for by industry trials is less than 10 percent, probably close to 7 percent. The PI estimates that hiring a full-time nurse costs $70,000 a year, including salary and fringe benefits. He continues: "Once you add the direct and indirect costs of the study you probably need to generate $100,000 to cover these costs, which at $5,000 per patient means that you need to enroll twenty patients. We average two to three patients a study. So you have to have probably eight to ten studies, so your nurse will be involved in eight to ten trials to generate her salary and we are not talking about benefits to CBTO. And eight to ten studies, two or three patients each . . . again, you have to understand that it is hard to enroll in these studies, so there is not much leverage. It's a hard business. So our studies, the studies we are doing at CBTO, are not self-sufficient, so the personnel involved to do these studies we have to pay them from other resources besides the resources we are generating from industry trials" (PI, 27 April 2004).

For the PI, the main reason why CBTO does trials is to bring a new agent or new treatment modality to patients who badly need one, or to answer a very important research question. "Let me give you an example, the SMART study is asking this very important question: once we start patients on treatment should we treat them for life or can we treat them as needed? And that is an important question."

COMPENSATION OF VOLUNTEERS IN HIV CLINICAL DRUG TRIALS

Not only does CBTO receive financial compensation for its participation in the trials but the volunteers themselves are often compensated for their enrollment, both in industry trials and also for the community-based research developed through the CPCRA. In contrast to phase I trials, in which subjects are paid hundreds or even thousands of dollars to join a trial, phases II, III, and IV offer considerably lower amounts. For example, SMART volunteers received $20 every four months. Industry trials offer similar financial benefits. Volunteers may also receive tokens or money to cover their parking expenses. According to the PI, financial compensation has become an indispensable part of clinical-trials research involving HIV drugs.

> Let me tell you one thing that unfortunately is reality. We cannot and unfortunately we will never be able to do [trials research] if the patient is not compensated to do these trials, unfortunately. Now, the problem we have, unless the trial is bringing something revolutionary to the table, patients are not very motivated, they have other choices, other therapeutic choices. Let's say you are trying to compare two regimes where the drugs have been FDA approved. The patient can get any of

these drugs without having to participate in the trial. If it is a new drug that is on the verge of being approved by the FDA and the patient feels that they might need this drug to survive then, they might do the study. So, it all depends on the need to do the trial. And even if there is a need to do the trial patients are not very motivated because they are taking time away from their work and spend a couple of hours every month or every two months and they need time for their travel, their parking, and sometimes need to be compensated for their time away from work. So compensation is becoming very important. It's a good incentive. (PI, 27 April 2004)

The PI seems to believe that willing HIV volunteers for drug trials have become a scare resource, one that needs to be lured back with financial incentives if industry trials are to continue. But maybe the scarcity of volunteers is less severe than the PI imagines. During the last ten years drug trials for HIV have multiplied to an unprecedented level while the HIV population has remained steady or nearly so. It may be that there is a shortage of volunteers partly because white males continue to be the standard for HIV trials nationwide, despite efforts by the NIH to incorporate women, African Americans, and Latinos into clinical trials. On the other hand, the PI is right in pointing out that many patients now have fewer incentives to join trials than in the past. Thanks to community mobilization and the collective action of AIDS organizations, through their health coverage HIV patients now have access to a wide range of therapeutic opportunities that simply were not present just ten years ago. This helps to explain why unless their lives are at stake or the trial is for a very promising drug, volunteers may hesitate to enter a trial and prefer to wait until the trial is completed and the drug is on the market.

The PI believes that the need to offer financial incentives to patients who join HIV trials presents an unintended consequence. He notes that patients who are supposed to enter the trial for altruistic reasons, or to help find a cure or improve a therapeutic option, end up joining the trial largely for the financial rewards, thus introducing a bias into the study. (I discuss the relationship between commodification in HIV trials research and research ethics in chapter 5.) "Ideally the patient should not be paid, and motivation should be the only reason to participate in a trial because you wanna answer the question, it's a scientific question that you want to answer, you understand the risks, you understand the benefits and you are not doing it for the money. Money might be a bias in a sense, but I think that we are not compensating them with money to save their lives, we are compensating them for parking. We compensate them for the toll they pay to cross the bridge. So, the compensation is symbolic, it's not gonna make them rich. Unfortunately some patients see it as a way to generate money and sometimes they get involved in trials they shouldn't be involved in—not in our site—but I read of patients doing things that they really shouldn't be doing" (PI, 27 April 2004).

5

HIV Clinical Trials and the Fight for Their Lives

THE STORIES OF JOHN, MICHAEL, AND GERALDINE

John, Michael, and Geraldine volunteered for HIV trials at CBTO. Michael is the only one to have volunteered for an industry trial, sponsored by Boehringer Ingelheim to test the efficacy of the drug Tipranavir, which is in the latest stages of development along with another drug from the same laboratory that was already approved. John and Geraldine were volunteering for a community trial, Wistar, although different versions of it. The trial did not involve drugs but was intended to assess the progress of the virus in certain patients. Since every trial offered financial compensation, I used these three cases to explore issues of financial compensation in relation to volunteers' participation in trials.

Like most volunteers for HIV trials at CBTO, John, Michael, and Geraldine are in their mid-forties. That two are male and one is female reflects the ratio prevailing among volunteers at CBTO as well as epidemiological trends in the United States. John and Geraldine are African American; Michael is white. This ratio also reflects the composition of CBTO patients, who are predominantly minority, in particular African American. Michael has a middle-class background while John and Geraldine, like the majority of CBTO's population, come from poorer families.

The narratives of these three volunteers allow us to understand their decisions to join a trial in more than an abstract sense by taking into account major biographical events in their lives and their present circumstances as they contend with HIV. Their experiences are quite different from those of the professional guinea pigs in phase I trials, but they offer insight into the extent of body commodification in later phases of drug research.

JOHN

When I met John he entered the office carrying a kid's bike he had found on the street on his way to CBTO. He was very happy about his find and hoped that although the bike was not in very good shape, he could still sell it and "make a buck." He had been living in a shelter and just recently managed to move to a rented room and live independently. John had been coming to the research department for years as a volunteer for the Wistar trial.

He was born in Augusta, Georgia, and came to Philadelphia when he was eighteen years old. John's father died when he was ten and he lived with his mom, older brother, and sister. He remembers that at school he always got good grades until the sixth grade, when he did a lot of drinking and drugs and got kicked back to grammar school. He regrets that he never learned to read. John started working very early in his life.

His father had a wood business, and when he died a friend of his bought his truck, coal, and everything else and John and his brother started working with him. This was his first job, out of necessity. "I've been always a survivor, you know what I mean? My mother didn't have enough money after my father died and she had to work and I had to learn how to cook at an early age if I wanted to eat. And back then you could sell soda bottles—they ain't got them here no more—I used to plug soda bottles to have extra money to go to the movies, to go to the football games on the weekends, it was a kind of hard struggle."

At sixteen John left Augusta to try his luck in Philadelphia, where his sister was living. He explained:

But for me, being the baby of the family, I was always experimenting and always kind of adventurous. I always wanted to try something new.

Like I said, I left Augusta at sixteen, quit the school, and got a job because I was curious, adventurous, and you know, Augusta is really small: at ten o'clock the bus stops running. If you live outside the city that means that you need a car. My sister, my older sister, lived in Philadelphia and she used to come down every Christmas and visit. So she said: "When do you come to Philadelphia?" Oh, yeah! I am wild anyway, you know what I mean. So I went, moved to Philadelphia in 1976, Ringle Street. I got a job later on that year at a restaurant called Geno's, I was eighteen. They sold burgers and they also sold Kentucky Fried Chicken, it was like two restaurants in one. So that was my first job here and I was cooking chicken. I catched real fast and the manager who hired me got real close.

When I came to Philadelphia I was just smoking weed but when I got here I got introduced to speed. I was doing speed on the job, me and my manager, I told him about it and he said: "bring me some in." He had never tried, he liked it, and we got real close. (John, 30 July 2004)

When John was working at the restaurant he met his future wife, who was also working there. "I met my wife in the same restaurant, we got a place together. I am still getting high, doing a lot of drugs, she was not but she didn't say anything because she was in love with me. We stayed together for two and a half years. I am working, she was working, but I would never stay home. She got pregnant and still I wouldn't be home but I was bringing money."

When something disappeared from the restaurant where he was working his friend and manager fired him. It was then that John, unemployed, started a career dealing drugs. "Then, I had a cousin that lived in Atlanta, whom I never met, and he started coming here bringing me pounds of weed. Now I am selling weed. I was walking around with $2,000 per day. He was coming like twice a week, bringing me weed. I am the king of the neighborhood now because, you know, back then weed was the real thing, like it is crack now but back then it was weed. I was living the life of Riley, everybody in the neighborhood giving me and my wife respect." It was around this time that John also started shooting speed. "I started using needles. One night I was with a couple of friends and they told me that I should try to shoot it and my being curious, adventurous, I did it. I couldn't hit myself so they did it and I tried and I liked it, so I started shooting it."

In 1979 John left his wife and started a relationship with a woman who was living across the street from his sister. After leaving his wife with two kids he went back to Atlanta. "My girl started tricking for money, you know. When I moved back to Atlanta I had another connection and I was selling weed. And this went on for years." After getting two tickets for driving under the influence John decided to go back to Philadelphia. He and his girlfriend moved in with her mother, the girlfriend went back to "tricking," and John found a job in a factory. "We were still doing our stuff," John told me, alluding to his drug habit, but then his girlfriend overdosed. "I was scared to shit. I put her in the bathtub in cold water and she came back." Although John was very much concerned about the risk of overdose from intravenous drug use, he was not aware of the risks of AIDS transmission. "Me and my girl, we shared needles, sure, I wasn't never too particular about it. I didn't hear about AIDS until the '90's. I was having sex wild, no condoms, nothing. So I was sharing needles a lot and sometimes they tell you that you need alcohol and bleach to clean it. But sometimes I just wait to whoever was taking the needles outside and run some water through it and dump it, but you can still see a little blood on the thing. That happened, I got HIV. I think that's the way I've got it because I know a lot of people with HIV now that I shared needles with. I could also have gotten it from unprotected sex because I never used condoms either. I still don't like them but I use them because they say that you can get locked up from spreading this shit. So I don't like them but I use them now."

After his girlfriend's last overdose she stopped using drugs and wanted John to stop as well. "I said: 'Why should I stop? I never OD.' But she wanted me to stop and then I went to Eagleville and had a seven-day blank. I got some pills, got caught and was kicked out. When my girlfriend saw me she told me 'What are you doing here? I thought you wanted to stop?' So, she kicked me out right away." Then John came back to Georgia and stayed at his mother's house in Augusta. He landed a job at a steel mill, "a damn good job, the highest-paying job I ever had." He worked there for two years but lost his job because of his drug use. "I was getting high too much, I couldn't get my ass to work. I got a job at another factory but that job, man, that job sucked. It was an animal food factory and the flies and the shit around sucked. All they do is change the name in the bag."

John was working when he learned that his mother had passed away. He then moved back with his older sister to Philadelphia. Shortly after returning to the city John went to jail after committing a crime to pay a drug-related debt, and there he learned that he had HIV. "And when I got locked up they do the test on me and that's how I knew I had HIV, 1998. I said: 'Why not do the test,' but I never thought I might have it. Before I knew I had it, I thought I would spread the shit then, then they will find a cure. But after I got it I changed my mind: no, I am not going to spread this shit, you know what I mean?"

MICHAEL

I met Michael when he came for a routine follow-up on an "industry trial." After living with HIV since the late 1980s he was running out of therapeutic options and hoped this new trial would give him new possibilities.

Michael was born in 1961 in Philadelphia. He had a middle-class upbringing. "Mother, father, one older sister. My dad was a chemist and my mom was a housemaker and a part-time worker. My childhood was somewhat dysfunctional. My father was an alcoholic, so that created a lot of distress in the family. I guess early childhood was OK. I wasn't a very happy child through my high school. I was questioning things in my teens and in high school, I was very uncomfortable and that led when I was fifteen or sixteen to a lot of marijuana usage. I think I was just trying to get away from a lot of stuff. That marijuana usage stopped after I flunked two years in high school, I had to do summer school, I quit smoking pot. I did well in high school" (Michael, 30 July 2004). After finishing high school Michael found a job in a restaurant in downtown Philadelphia. He frequented gay places downtown but struggled with his sexual identity. "I am in a struggle there because, as I said, I am almost eighteen and I still haven't quite figured this out. I never had a sexual experience until downtown. I associate being homosexual with failure, that is what I was told. Failure in not fitting in, in being different. I was very concerned about it in my job. I've worked with a lot of gay individuals and I loved them all, very much, I wasn't ready to come out yet. Early on there was a lot of, you know, sitting on the fence for fear. I associate success with being straight."

At twenty, wanting to "fit in," Michael left the restaurant business and went to work in the credit department of a bank while still taking part-time courses to get an accounting degree. He engaged heavily in anonymous sex and binge drinking.

I wanted a "regular job." I stayed there. Now, my drinking is escalating a lot with a lot of binge drinking. I was coming downtown—still living in Northeast—and a lot of, you know, the cinema . . . I wasn't going a lot to gay bars. I was just doing a lot of anonymous sex. That lasted for a while and then finally I met a guy and I guess I felt in love and I was still living at home but things were securing up with my mom and then I thought that it was time to leave. I was twenty-three. It was right in the '80s, '83, '84, that time. At that time I still had a boyfriend downtown. He was fifteen years older than I was, very nice. He was doing fine but he hadn't come out either. Even I came out before he did. In our relationship he was not out in public. By the time I was twenty-four I had finally done that.

I also decided that I wanted to cook. I loved the bank but I decided that it was time to pursue a cooking career. If I was going to do it at any time, it was there. I went to the Restaurant School here in Philadelphia and I embarked on that. So I am in a new apartment alone, totally new job—I went to work to the Fish Market Restaurant—and I worked full-time night and I went to school full-time day. I was really burning up fast. Between that year and the drinking I know I killed myself.

Things were going very well, working, studying, living alone, but it was a year of madness, very lonely, very lonely. I had no connections with downtown. Even when I met people I knew from the bars I was really at a loss. And with all the sex that had been going on, all this madness.

By the mid-1980s the HIV epidemic was already under way, and Michael could not avoid taking note. "I remember watching the TV one time and channel 4 had this thing and it really hit me. I guess it was 1987 by now, it was a special and it had two guys talking on the phone. It was a play focused on AIDS and it was a presentation of an off-Broadway show that ran in New York. So I remember watching it, I focus on these two guys talking on the phone, very sad, back and forth talking about a friend. And you hear that and you know that it's happening around here and in San Francisco and it was like the second or third time that I ask myself this question. I wish I hadn't done anything wrong, but I knew I had. I knew it was a problem. But when I saw the TV piece I thought, I wish I hadn't done anything, poured another drink, and thought: "Well, let's see what happens." I wonder if I had met anybody in the restaurant business with AIDS. I definitely heard of people passing away but I was trying to shut it off."

Despite Michael's efforts to "shut off" the risk of HIV transmission, two years later he was forced to deal with his own status as HIV-positive.

So, I came down with hepatitis B. This might have been early '89. Mid-'89 I was sick as a dog. I was so sick and I had no health insurance, I had no doctor—I was working but with no health insurance—and really blind to the gay man's disease. Except for the usual sexual diseases I was ignorant of all that. I was not even addressing things and it was crazy. I am paying for it dearly now. I called my sister and she called Jefferson. And the nurse-administrator set me up with the doctor. The guy was a very nice guy, probably the greatest guy in the world. So, he needs to see me. I go back that same day and he was waiting for me. I could barely walk, I was so sick. He laid me down and told me that they were doing the bloodwork and that they would call me as soon they came in. I had the idea that I might have HIV in the back of my mind but not really. He suggests an HIV test and I thought, "OK, you have to do what you have to do." He brings me back and then he gives me my HIV diagnosis so now I am really like a wreck. Everything was a mess. I thought my life was over. I was only twenty-eight years old and I thought that I was just gonna die. He told me: "You are gonna go five years." My doctor said: "This is what we do for this, this is how we treat this. You feel very sick now. It's probable that is the hepatitis. I've seen your counts and based on this you probably had this for two years because your counts are at 300. That means that you have had this for a while. I am gonna give you five years. You are gonna have five years.

GERALDINE

Geraldine was introduced to me by Grace, the head nurse in the research department. Geraldine had been coming to CBTO as a patient first, then engaged in weekly women's support groups and finally ended up working as a peer-educator coordinator. In her mid-forties, she was born in Hawaii but did not stay there for long. Her father was in the navy, which forced the family to move frequently, until her parents got divorced and she moved with her mother and brothers to Delaware.

I had two brothers, one younger and one older than me. I was seven and I was in Delaware until I was seventeen years old. I went to kindergarten and first grade in California, second grade in Delaware, and I graduated from high school there.

While I was in high school I started doing marijuana and doing drugs and drinking, you know, the high school kid kind of stuff. So then I moved on to doing cocaine when I was in my twenties. In 1983 I had one child, I graduated when he was six months.

I was living with my son's father for a little while and he didn't want to support us. I had a little job here and there. I was seventeen. I worked at Campbell's soup factory and then I worked in King Cole, another factory. At Campbell's I was sorting vegetables all day and King Cole was the same way but it was a clam factory and I had to sort the clams from the shells, I liked that job. It's just a small, little piece that you pull out, with your fingers. It came already open. Then I worked at Thompson, which is a chicken factory, but I just lasted thirty days. In the chicken factory I had to grab the chicken's kidney and stuff and all up to here [the arm], my wrist would be so sore after the day because I had to grab it and you had to do like two at a time. So I didn't last that job too long. Then I tried to do some job training but it didn't work. And then I started using drugs heavily and then at twenty-three, twenty-four I moved to Wilmington, Delaware. I just moved there because I went to jail for shoplifting in Dover so I spend there like six months and then they put me on work release and I had a little job doing janitorial work. (Geraldine, 2 August 2004)

After being released from jail Geraldine stopped using drugs for a while, then resumed her drug use and engaged in prostitution to afford the drugs and shelter. It was then that she was arrested for prostitution by an undercover police officer and went back to jail for six months. Some time after she was released Geraldine came back to jail once more, also on prostitution charges. About this time she found out that she had HIV.

Somewhere in between I found out I was HIV-positive, it was 1989 when I was diagnosed. I just had a cold that I could not get rid of and it was this time of year, August, and I couldn't shake this cold. So I went to the doctor and he said that he would treat me for the cold but that he wanted to do an HIV test. And me: "Sure, go ahead, if you have to take it, you have to take it. Do it." Not thinking that it would come out positive. I never thought about it. Even when I was sharing needles and stuff I never thought about it because I was trying to get high. And also they didn't have much education at Wilmington, they only had bleach kits and condoms, that was the outreach. And that's as far as the street outreach went. They didn't say that you constantly do these things, that you always have to have bleach kits and all the stuff, they never said that. They just gave us a bleach kit and condoms and that was it. They never sit down with us and explain things to us. I never knew anybody with HIV, nothing, nobody. I never asked, and back then you couldn't tell because you didn't look like you had HIV. So when I found out I was upset, I was four months clean and I started using again because the doctor said: "You have AIDS and you are gonna die." He didn't say go to this place to get medical care, or there are these help groups, no.

COPING WITH HIV

Once he learned about his HIV John equated his diagnosis with a death sentence, an assumption made by many health workers, patients, and the public alike in the 1980s. However, a few years later his contact with Action AIDS, a community-based organization, led him to reevaluate his situation.

I didn't know that much about it and I thought: "Damn, I am dying." I know that they have no cure, then I am dying. But after I thought a little more about it if you take your medication you can live a normal life. My case manager told me these things. Because when I was in jail Action AIDS comes to jail, so I had a case manager. And they put me in another cell with other people with HIV, everybody in the house was HIV. And they had a lot of meetings, told me about HIV, that it's not a killer, that having HIV is not AIDS, well, I got educated. Still not sinking in: I got HIV, how the hell I did that? I should have been more careful but I didn't give a fuck.

When I learned that I had HIV then, a couple of friends of mine which were shooting drugs told me they were HIV. I never told nobody. The only people I told I was HIV is my family.

John not only received information about HIV and became more confident about the outcomes but also managed to receive treatment from a top medical doctor and researcher from a local university. "The doctor I am hooked up with now, I've been with him for four years. He worked at Temple and he moved to Presbyterian, he is the chief of the infectious disease department. So I have one of the top doctors in the country. He goes all over the country giving presentations and stuff. I just stick with him and I stopped using drugs for a while. I stopped using drugs about one year and a half because I am still trying to figure this shit out. I am going to tell people about my HIV or not? I am going to tell a girl I am with that I am HIV even when I am using a condom? Why should I tell her?"

John kept going to Action AIDS regularly and this past year started working with them on outreach among male shelter residents.

> I meet my case manager every week at Action AIDS. Now I am a volunteer. They have this new program and I have my little cards I pass out. I've been working for over a month now and I gave out more than four hundred cards in shelters, drop-in centers where people came from all over the country and they have nowhere to go. I give them cards to go and get tested for AIDS. They get counseling and shelter, the same thing I got. What we are trying to do is to have them to come in. The cards have my last four digits of my social security card and last week just eight people showed up, so I know it was me. I want to spread the world that you can get tested and still have a normal life before it is too late. Well, no, I wouldn't say a normal life because I feel different now. My life changed because, you know, I heard people talking about other people who got HIV and it's like they got plague or something. Like, if I touch you, you might get HIV; they don't know but that's what they think. I hear people talking about people who I know they have HIV and I don't want them to talk about me like that. And I just got out of a relationship with this girl—she got HIV and she was my first HIV partner—and she told me right away. I didn't told her that I had it: she read it on my medication. She was kind of calm about it. I came late that night and she said: "Why didn't you tell me that you had HIV?" and I: "Uh? How do you know?" She said: "Why are you taking these medications? I've seen your medicine." "So, I got it too. OK, all right." This is recent, this is, like, two weeks she stayed with me.

John is currently taking HIV medication and doing well. He told me that since he cannot read the drug names he knows which ones to take by looking at their colors. The system works fine for him, and he hasn't missed a dose. "I saw my doctor and he said that I don't need to start taking medication right away. Like I said, I have a top doctor in the field. Then I said: 'Well, doctor it's up to you,' and he said, 'Right now everything is cool.' Then I said: 'OK, let's start taking the medication.' I started talking with [CBTO's phlebotomist] and she knows I am taking my medication, because every time she do my blood draw everything is undetected, I have no problem taking my medication. I get my pills once a month and I am getting them religiously, you know what I mean? I don't miss a dose, I take them twice a day. I haven't missed a dose in four years."

After being diagnosed Michael learned that he had five years more to live. He started taking AZT, the only drug available at that time, kept working, and stepped up his alcohol consumption.

> You probably are gonna get sick during these five years and we are gonna take care the best we can. But I cannot guarantee you a comfortable life after five years. He said: think about that. I am twenty-eight, so this is not good. He said that he would keep me as comfortable as possible and that I would be under his care, don't worry about anything. And he started me on AZT. Then he stopped it because my counts had gone up and then he tried again with AZT when the count went down. And that began the process. That was the initial drug.

> I went back to work. I was determined. I just forgot about the five-year plan, I blocked it out. I took the AZT, I drunk more vodka, and I got another job. I had a new job and then I had to address the HPB so I had to go into a surgery for that. So I took care of that and I was like in a lot of pain for that and I thought: "What have I done?" I was a wreck. I was really a train wreck. I just still worked hard and I just kept going.

Around that time Michael also met someone with whom he started a relationship and moved in. He also kept working in the restaurant business. "I met a guy—in one of these obscure places—but I liked the guy and he was older than me, divorced. And the thing was that he accepted me for what I had. Because I had a lot of rejection, even in a few months I was not having . . . so, we went into a relationship very early on. We were happy initially. I entered for all the wrong reasons: for acceptance because I felt that I couldn't do any better. So, we got together, it should be 1990 then, I moved him in and I continued to work." At work and outside his close circle Michael attempted to hide his HIV diagnosis. "Remember people were dying by then. I am noticing it, my eyes were just more open to the whole idea. Not really friends but I see co-workers I am noticing this rumor, and this and that, a lot of gossip and rumor and crap. Because I was trying to hide my diagnosis so I was trying to hide the pills and stuff, you know.

"I still worked—I don't know how, it's just amazing—my T cell count was 180, so there was always back and forth to the doctors. I had lung problems but I would just keep going. That's what I did. I just keep running back and forth between doctors and they keep treating me. It was either a false alarm or if they got it, they got it and then I came back to do my things."

Michael continues taking AZT, holds on, keeps working, and becomes more knowledgeable about resources for HIV patients. He also keeps fighting opportunistic infections and his longtime alcohol habit.

At that point I was still managing, right now we are at the point where it is AZT and d4T. There aren't a lot of drugs out there, '91, '92, it was right at that point where if you didn't catch the proteases you would die. So I hang on for a while with that and then I went to . . . it's kind of a blur because I am such an alcoholic mess at that time. I went back to work at that time and I was just trying to keep my head above water, to maintain financial independence, things like that, pay the health insurance, the AZT was covered by the State of Pennsylvania and what have you. So I was also getting knowledgeable about drugs and the SPBP and all the good stuff but I was always in a state of high anxiety with the whole thing. At around that time, in '93, I got another job with a big catering service and I worked for them, it was good, it was a good thing. But at this point I am not feeling well, I had another herpes outbreak. My boss protected me, I think that she knew what was going on. I cannot remember if I told her or not. I probably did and I have a feeling that she didn't care, she was OK with it. I kept working, '93, and then I started to have a breakdown. Checked myself in an institution to come off of the alcohol but that was unsuccessful— stayed for a while but I even got drunk inside. I went back to work but fell on the stairs. They gave me unemployment and vacation time: "When you are ready to come back, you come back." They were so nice. I was less healthy. I couldn't get into a clinical trial for protease inhibitors because my T cell count was too low, my doctor was very concerned and I sort of started to give up.

With his health deteriorating, Michael decided to retire from the restaurant business and file for disability. "So, I filed for disability in 1994—I regret that now—it was advised at that point. I just had three hearings, no attorney, I did everything on my own, did everything I had to do and they granted it. So I stayed home, went to volunteer at Jefferson, I drank heavily, and I kind of existed for a number of years under that. I had a pair of little jobs doing catering, nothing so steady. It was a life of just decadence and debauchery. No stable relationship, just myself and the house and I moved a roommate in. We existed for a while, didn't work, so he left, I brought another in and for a period of '93 to '95 I stayed in the house with roommates."

Around the mid-1990s the first protease inhibitors become available through expanded access programs, and Michael did not miss the opportunity:

At that point Crixivan had just arrived—or Fortovase?—the first one. So then I quickly went to expanded access and started it right away. I didn't do the trials, my T cell counts were too low to do the trials. They wanted people with higher counts. But this drug was available and before it was in pharmacies I was getting it. So I started on a protease inhibitor as soon as it came out. I was probably on AZT, Epivir, DdI, there wasn't a whole lot. I was on a combination and I made it over the hump. I wasn't feeling good, the drugs were like the worst. Also what happens is that I was getting sick from liver disease now because of my alcoholism. I had complicated everything with my alcoholism, so I had a bad liver and my doctors were very, very concerned. And about 1994 I had extended liver damage, my T cells were dropping like crazy, I was even trying not to drink for periods of time. I knew about AA but I wasn't easy to go there because I wanted to drink. So, I kept that way, I finally lost the house because I couldn't keep up with the payment so I moved from there to a little apartment across the street, where I am right now. That was 1995. I was still seeing David occasionally, he would come by, we had sex sometimes—behind his boyfriend's back—typical madness.

And all this time I had been case-managed through Jefferson and also Action AIDS. All the expanded program access I did it on my own. My doctor and myself did it. I felt like I had all the time in the world to do paperwork, so I did.

In the spring of 1996 Michael tried for the first time to stop drinking by enrolling in Alcoholics Anonymous. He did not stay in the program for long and his health deteriorated. Despite his troubles, ten years after being diagnosed Michael started to realize that he might "make it over the hump."

I didn't stay in that AA meeting. I moved into the apartment in '95, I went to the first AA meeting on my own in spring of '96. At this point the alcohol had destroyed my hip, had destroyed my liver, my count was low, I couldn't walk, I needed to use a cane, it just had gotten ridiculous. So, I went, stayed ten, fifteen days, drunk again, but it was tempting.

I filed for bankruptcy in '97, tried to clean some of the wreckage. I was always seeking the new drugs that were coming up, I was always seeking into whatever was happening. I was still being taken care by the doctors over Jefferson. I was always coming with infections and stuff and they did a fantastic job. Everything that seemed to come out of me they seemed to treat. I was always getting one fucking thing after another and I was always sick. This was ten years after I was diagnosed, pretty amazing, absolutely! The sprinkles were one of the worst because they were all over your face and people could see it, I was thinking: "this is not happening to me." But the doctors took great care of me.

I had specialty HIV care at Jeff, not a particular doctor yet, we switched over. More of the protease drugs started coming on the market at that point, '97—I am not sure. I started Crixovan right away and I started thinking that maybe I would make it over the hump here. I started thinking that I could do it, that I would get through this mess. But now, I was a full-blown-up alcoholic and I had been for a long time.

That year Michael tried again to curb his alcohol habit and went back to AA. This time he succeeded.

I started to go to AA and I stayed. 1997 to mid-'98, that year was not nice. Not real wreckage. In that year I got more time sober than I ever did and then in '99 I just stopped. I stayed in AA and became part of it, I broke off with everybody from outside, all ties. So, now is what I do. I focus my life on that. I will be sober six years in January this year. I had the five-year coin. So what I do is that I spend a lot of time on that, I volunteer in the community center so I am back more in gay life than I have ever been—than I was when I was drinking. I am more involved in the community, instead of just a bar. I volunteered in Washington West project which is an HIV testing site, on Locust, right on the block. I've volunteered for two or three years and that was a very good experience for me. So I guess it's pretty much it. I guess I am happier, not dating right now but I still struggle around being with guys that are positive, I am not sure whether I am gonna go with that. I met a couple of guys at AA but I am hesitant, I don't want to destroy that thing, you know? He is negative, I am positive but also he is recently ill. I think that maybe it is too much too soon. It's crazy out there, there are always a couple of guys coming to the meetings recently diagnosed.

When Geraldine learned about her HIV status she had been in and out of jail and also in and out of rehabilitation programs for her drug addiction. She tried to ignore her HIV status and did not change her lifestyle for some time. Then she found a support group for people living with HIV.

I found out about this support through my addiction because I went to a rehab for drugs and alcohol and my counselor told me about support groups for people living with HIV. But I still wanted to get high, so I went to that group but they knew that when I didn't come was because I was getting high and they would come for me and they would miss me for two or five minutes but they still would come for me because, you know, it was that kind of support group. No, I never thought about becoming HIV-positive. Why I was trying to get clean for? So I thought that I was enjoying by myself—that's what I thought I was doing, enjoying by myself—kept doing the same stuff, no protection, nothing. I kept doing that until I was pregnant with my daughter and then I didn't know who the father was because I was still tricking and all that stuff. I had unprotected sex, of course, and I didn't believe in abortions —I never had and I never had an abortion—so had her and she's been blessed because she is not HIV-positive. I was more concern about her than myself because they retested me again, but this time when I got the results I was at the doctor's office at an infectious disease clinic. They sat me down and explained to me everything. They told me that I should go there for my medical care, they just came out with AZT so there was more hope from the first diagnosis when they told me that in a couple of years I was gonna die. Which back then, it was true, I guess, but I am still here. When I went out I started tricking and stuff and my daughter ended up in foster care in Delaware. Then, when I really realized that I really wasn't going to die it's when I decided to change. Around late '92, I was still doing drugs and stuff but I was still here. So I thought, they told me two years and I am still here, they lied to me. So when I realized that I was still here I thought that I had to do something because I had two children already.

It was then that Geraldine decided that she wanted to stop using drugs, but she needed to enroll in a rehab drug program. "So what I did is that I saw my counselor and we did another assessment for me to go inpatient. So three months later my counselor calls me. I am still getting high but the last day was May 15, tried to get high but didn't have more money and instead of going out I stayed in bed. The next day my counselor calls me saying I had a bed. I was ready for it. I stayed in the program for one year and then outpatient for another year." Free of her drug habit, Geraldine turned to the HIV women's support group managed by Action AIDS.

Then I started going to HIV support groups. I got hooked up with Action AIDS, they had a women's support group, then I went to another support group in Dinn Street, that was for everybody, that was co-ed, and then I started getting educated about the disease and then I started peer education—'95 or '96 is when I did my first presentation to children about HIV/AIDS in a community center, and I was explaining about AZT and everything related to drugs. It was fun and they got a lot of information from me. Then I started doing more presentations through the speakers of Action AIDS. Then at Action AIDS we did a program called Woman-to-Woman program, then I started the Project Teach at CBTO in '97. Then I got offered a position here in 2000 as assistant case manager. March 2001 they asked me if I wanted the position of outreach person, by March of the following year they asked me to be case manager assistant. I am also studying but it is frustrating. I didn't even have time to do my financial aid for the fall semester yet, so I am trying to get that done. But I didn't have time because my husband has mental health issues. We are getting away for this weekend so we don't have to do anything.

I started taking medication for AIDS in July '97. My first cocktail was Sequanavir, AZT, D50, and Napavir. That lasted until October '97 and then it was Crixovan, Epivir, and Zerit, I took that for, like, seven years. Now I am on Ziagen, Viramune, and Viread.

One of the things the three informants have in common, besides their initial denial of HIV, their struggles with drug and alcohol addiction, and their precarious lifestyles, is their encounter with AIDS community organizations that gave them new insight into the meaning and perspectives of being HIV-positive. Through this interaction they gained valuable information about the disease, their prognosis, and possible treatments—which increased during the 1990s, in particular after 1995. This participation empowered them to keep fighting and gave them new spaces in which to find support they needed. All got involved in community-based organizations and participated in meetings and their organizational or outreach activities. John even managed to get some financial support by doing outreach work, and Geraldine became a professional HIV peer educator.

HIV TRIALS AND THE FIGHT FOR THEIR LIVES

John's contact with CBTO was initially through a study he was doing sponsored by Presbyterian, the hospital of the University of Pennsylvania. Although John is not sure what the trial is designed for, he knows that he can monitor his viral load and have access to valuable information about the workings of the virus. He is on a fixed income, and the financial compensation helps him to make ends meet.

My doctor at Presbyterian introduced me to somebody at Presbyterian but it was done here at CBTO. Before I dealt with CBTO's phlebotomist I met three or more people but she is the nicest one. I don't know exactly what are they looking for when they draw the blood, but the only thing I know is that I have to have my blood drawn anyway to see my viral load and stuff. So, they was giving money to draw my blood, why not take it? I am on a fixed income, you know what I mean? My case manager just did a money budget for me, what I pay and what I am getting. I came $200 over what I get because I smoke cigarettes.

Cigarettes is $5, five times thirty, that's a lot of money. I have to pay for my room and I don't get food stamps, so I have to buy my food and I like to eat; food ain't cheap. With HIV you have to try to maintain a diet, you have to eat vegetables and stuff. So it's kind of rough to survive, man, but I am a survivor. I was a survivor since I was sixteen. I'm on my own.

I get a check from disability, four hundred and eighty something, and I am getting a check from the flyers of $124 once a month. Together that's $611, that ain't nothing. Then, occasionally, my sister has a neighbor and if I wash up her car, that's $20. And sometimes I do odd jobs, a neighbor wants me to go to the store. It's rough but I am going to make it. I do whatever to survive.

John receives a check for disability and uses welfare programs for access to medication and health care.

I am still on welfare for the medication, I have insurance. I have all the medicine I need for free, that's one good thing about them. Not in all the United States, but in Philadelphia they see that you get your medication but it's different for different states. Like, in Georgia a man cannot get on welfare, only a woman and she has to got kids. If you cannot make it in Philadelphia you cannot make it nowhere because there are so many places with benefits, all you need to do is walk a little to get it but it's worth it. And I am an independent guy, I am on my own. While I did the shelter thing, I don't like nobody telling me what to do, when to go to sleep. So, I told to myself, the money I was fucking up doing drugs and shit: that's the place to stay. So I quit. I said, I take that money and put it in a place to stay. So for the last two years I've been on my own, out of drugs and I have my own place, you know what I mean? I am paying bills again—I haven't been paying bills for so long—I am gonna get telephone bills, I am paying light bills, water bills. I need a phone, you know, in case something might happen at night and my sister be worry about me and shit. She comes twice a month, unless something happens. I know I should visit her more. Yes, I need a phone. I am gonna get a phone next week.

Since being diagnosed as HIV-positive in the mid-1980s Michael had been under medical treatment, and as a result he had exhausted almost all drug regimens. He came to CBTO a few months ago to enroll in a trial, hoping that it could bring new therapeutic options for him.

I decided to do this trial at CBTO because we sort of ran out of options because I always have this high resistant type because I did so many things and some of them are cousins of cousins. My doctor said: "You are doing OK but I don't have anything else to give you." He is at Jefferson but he knew about Zanavir so he set me up with Mark Walkings because he had early access but he pulled a genotype out of me and said: "Don't even bother to take it, it will fail, fail, fail," and we believed him in the end. So between him and my doc we moved into other options. What about a T20 trial coming into place? But I missed it because the T-cell count was different. They wanted fifty and under and I was above that, so I missed it. So then they wanted to send me to Belleview because they didn't have anything left. He said: "I can run just one more oral with you and then we are out of options. We need to find some options to back you up for these five more years." My doctor called me and said: "You know I really want you to consider CBTO." He really had wanted to consider CBTO a long time ago but now he said it was the time: "It's here, it's coming, you have to go," and I said OK. That's how I appeared here. And at the same time I started looking at T20. We got expanded access for that. Now I am taking T20, Tipranavir, Norvir, Tricevir, Viriad. Basically four drugs in the same class and then T20—his own—and then Tipranavir and Norvir is part of the clinical trial. So you have all the classes covered, except for the middle class, which I am done with that. Previously I've tried a drug with my doctor by Giulliard called Previard. It was supposed to be another nuke but it was a failure.

This trial seems to be working for Michael, helping him to cope better. The trial along with the medication he is receiving "creates a better life" for him.

I feel very happy with this trial. I have some problems with the orals now, it's been a while but I have some stomach distress lately and I have to address that. Also, the needle was OK but there wasn't a lot of fat that I had, so right now I am concentrating the needles on the belly, so 99 percent of my needles go in here. It's hard to push the needle but it gets in there.

For Tipranavir and T20 I get expanded access. As long as the drug doesn't kill anybody I think they are gonna keep it in expanded access. For all purposes I plan to stay on T20, Norvir, and Tipranavir for as long as I can take them. My numbers are much better now. I never had a viral load under one or two million. The lowest I had was 60,000 and now it is undetectable. This is the first time in my life. One little, tiny time I had it with Crixivan but it lasted a month and then it fell apart. If the viral load comes down, the pain goes down, it's weird. I used to wake up in the morning and I couldn't move, the overall physical pain had gotten really bad and it's funny how that has changed. That's one thing researchers should start asking and researching about. So it does create a better life.

Michael is dependent on a disability check and finds his financial situation tight, but he manages with the help of a supportive family. Feeling better and more confident, he intends to find a part-time administrative job. "I go over my budget nearly 75 dollars a month. I am going over $1,000 in debt a year. It's not bad. My family is generous but not wealthy. My mom helps me out, a fifty, a hundred here, Christmas time. So it's good, I have a supporting family, they love me, if I ever go into financial trouble they bail me out but I always try to live within these $800 a month. I'm feeling it's time to get a legal part-time job, like receptionist, similar to what I do in the community center, I answer phones, etc."

Geraldine entered the Wistar trial in December. The trial does not involve any drug test but rather assessed variations in viral load.

I am doing the Wistar trial here and I am still on medication. The first part of the study was that they were drawing blood every month and when I became undetectable they would draw blood for like two more times and they would, after eight, sixteen, no thirty-two weeks would draw your blood for the last time but they still would see you. My next time I will have my blood draw will be September. I am not getting any new medication in this trial, I take my own meds. I started it in December. I wanted to help other people, not just me.

I am getting my medication through SPBP, a state program developed through the Department of Public Welfare for people who work whose income is not over $30,000 a year. If you work and have a higher income you then have other options. Medicines are high. In '97 I was getting my medication through medical assistance. But as I started working more hours I lost that and I got this one last year. If you are not working you can apply for SPBP but you can also apply for medical assistance.

Currently Geraldine is working, trying to finish an associate's degree in drug counseling, and taking care of three children and her ailing husband.

Right now I am living with my husband and three of my children. After I entered my last rehab program I found I was pregnant with my last child. They had AZT for the mother, monitored the baby, and that was it. But they kept me on my medicines until I entered labor. They gave me a Cesarean. This is April 1993 and the doctor says: "If he is not breathing I am not trying to save him." "How can he say something like that—he is an African doctor?" I said to myself, I am not going to worry about that. When I saw him breathing, ah, ah, ah, that's it! Henry is like his father. He's a miracle, he shouldn't be here. My thirteen-years-old daughter came home April 4th, on her birthday [from foster care] nine years ago. And then my baby son is six. All different personalities, my personality, their personalities, oh, my goodness!

I think that I had more money before I started working. I am broke just a few days after payday and I didn't use to be broke a few days after payday. Now I have to pay all these bills, we have to buy our food because we don't get food stamps because we are getting too much money. I am not getting a check from disability because I work. Before I had received checks but now I don't because I work. My husband gets disability. He has arthritis in both ankles. He cannot walk outside the house.

I think that it's good that other people that are HIV-positive to look at life a little bit different and know that just because they have HIV that doesn't mean that they cannot work, they cannot do things for themselves, because they can. I am struggling sometimes but it can be done.

A COMMON THEME IN THE NARRATIVES: BEING A SURVIVOR

Despite their differences of gender, class, race, and sexual orientation, the life stories of John, Michael, and Geraldine reveal similar trajectories. That they are aware and proud of their ability to hold on, to struggle, to survive, to make it in very difficult circumstances is hard to miss in their accounts. The notion of struggling and their self-perception as survivors not only structures their accounts but shapes their identities, allowing them to make sense of their past and their present as HIV patients and trial participants.

For all three the trial is one more strategy for coping with the disease. To Michael it offers the possibility of testing new drugs in their last stages of development that have not been introduced to the market yet, expanding his already limited therapeutic options.

For John and Geraldine, who are doing better with their HIV conditions, the trial is not a life-and-death matter but instead offers them the possibility of contributing to the development of scientific knowledge while also gaining valuable information about their health and the workings of the virus. It is clear that for these patients trials offer empowerment by making them active participants in their struggle against AIDS. Knowing their viral loads, or knowing how the body responds to the virus, offers a sense of agency and control. But there seems to be an additional gain from participating in trials. Geraldine, John, and Michael have experienced an improvement in their quality of life.

This perception is confirmed by the PI, who suggests that patients who are enrolled in trials tend to do better than those who are not:

> It's my impression that patients that are involved in trials tend to do better than patients that are not involved in trials, in general. And the reason is that being involved in trials, they are monitored very closely, they have more support, they are closely monitored, there is that accountability that goes on, the regular visits, and every time a patient shows up for his visits he is reminded that it is extremely important that he takes the medication, getting five, six calls in between visits from the study coordinating to see how he is doing, reminding him to take his medication, stuff like that. And for definition, when somebody gets involved in a trial, understanding what the commitment is he has to really make to be in a trial, that tells you something about the background of the patient. These are usually those who care, who are very obsessive, they want to really do everything right. But nevertheless, being in studies is important because it really keeps the patient involved. We still have problems of adherence. Sometimes we have

people that come with the bottle half-full. And we tell them, why are you not taking your medication? But again, the fact that they are coming regularly to see their doctor is helpful. The number of visits in a trial is more common than non-trial patients. We see our patients usually four times a year. If they are in a trial they have to come eight to nine times a year.

Finally, for some patients there is an additional, financial gain. This played a role in John's and Geraldine's decision to enter the trial, even if it was not their main one. For Michael, who had a larger support network and help from family, as well as higher stakes in the outcome of the trial, financial compensation was not relevant.

The attitudes of Geraldine, John, and Michael toward financial compensation reflect similar views among the larger population of patients enrolled in HIV trials at CBTO. Two-thirds of respondents to a semi-structured survey that I did among volunteers mentioned helping science to find a cure or to improve treatment options as their only motive for joining a trial, while some expressed their hope that the trial would benefit them therapeutically as well. For the remaining one-third of the volunteers surveyed, financial compensation was a factor in their decision. Yet these respondents may have been motivated by serious financial need. Unlike the professional guinea pigs taking part in earlier phases of drug development, volunteers for HIV trials at CBTO do not perceive themselves as a commodities, trading their bodies for financial gain. They see themselves as patients and are treated as such by the researchers and staff.

The narratives of the volunteers who are the focus of this chapter suggest that all three perceive themselves as survivors who have overcome very difficult circumstances. Their struggle to survive pushed them to get educated about their disease, take an active role that included participating in AIDS organizations, and searching for medical resources, among which they count their decision to join the HIV trials. Although all are grateful for the money earned in the trials, financial motivations are not primary. Instead they see the trials as an opportunity to empower themselves in their fight against the disease, a way to take control of their bodies and their lives.

6

FROM PRISONERS TO PROFESSIONALS

A Brief History of the Clinical-Trial Enterprise

> It is not possible nowadays to do any kind of clinical trial without some
> kind of financial compensation to volunteers for their participation.
> —CBTO PRINCIPAL INVESTIGATOR

Conducting clinical trial drug research in America today involves the
financial compensation of human subjects for their participation. The
differences regarding subjects' financial compensation are striking. In
some cases volunteers get a few hundred dollars, in others thousands.

And it is not only the subjects who are compensated by entering the
clinical trial economy. Researchers and research sites receive financial
compensation as well. According to Marcia Angell, a medical doctor
might receive $7,000 for enrolling a patient in a trial, and this sum can
increase, as doctors receive bonuses for fulfilling quotas. Angell criticizes
this commodification of the clinical-trials enterprise, arguing that it creates a conflict of interest between doctors and researchers on the one
hand and their patients on the other, while also negatively influencing
the outcome of the trials (Angell 2004).

According to Center Watch, an information services company that
monitors clinical research, there were more than eighty thousand clinical
trials being conducted in 2002 in America alone. Impressive as these
figures are, they represent only a fraction of the total number of trials
being conducted globally. Since 1980 the pharmaceutical industry, looking to speed the drug approval process and operating in an environment
of increasingly concentrated and globalized clinical-trials drug research,

has shipped many clinical trials abroad, mainly to developing countries where ethical regulations are more relaxed, nonexistent, or unenforced, and where a large population of willing, poor, disenfranchised subjects enter the trials, induced by the prospect of getting access to health care, drugs, and medical supervision, as well as financial rewards (Petryna 2005; Petryna 2009).

This chapter describes some major points leading to the commodification of human subjects' participation in pharmaceutical clinical-trials research in America, focusing on two related phenomena. The first is the shift from clinical trials using captive populations to populations recruited on the open market. This shift brought about changes in the social organization of clinical trials, particularly the emergence of "controlled experiment designs" involving different types of knowledge based on modern statistical techniques and new institutional arrangements to implement them. The second phenomenon is the historical development of the pharmaceutical industry in Philadelphia, beginning around 1970 and continuing until the present, as the city has seen its industrial economy replaced by one based on services and especially biomedical research and medical services. Toward the end of this chapter I document how these shifts affected people at the lower levels of the social structure by creating a reserve army of human research subjects.

FROM INSTITUTIONALIZED SUBJECTS TO THE MARKET RECRUITMENT OF PAID SUBJECTS

Scientific research involving human subjects was conducted until relatively recently on captive populations, without formal ethical procedures. Usually the research subjects came from the lower strata of society: the poor and the disenfranchised, sometimes recruited from orphanages, mental hospitals, and prisons. General hospital wards often provided poor, unaware subjects for scientific experimentation. Although the majority of research subjects were underprivileged, sometimes medical students and their teachers volunteered to be research subjects as well (Altman 1998).

Although formal ethical guidelines were lacking, the situation was not a free-for-all. According to Lereder, the law already protected human subjects from the effects of negligence. And the most general canons of medical ethics defined the professional duties of medical doctors toward their patients. The Hippocratic Oath, for example, requires physicians not to harm the patients during treatment. In addition, researchers had the responsibility to obtain the consent of their patients before subjecting them to experimental treatments (Lereder 1995). In 1940 the American Medical Association established guidelines to obtain the informed consent of patients who volunteered for biomedical research.

Marks points to the same requirement concerning patients participating in clinical trials during the Second World War (Marks 1997). However, no formalized procedures to obtain informed consent were established at that time, and the responsibility for seeking consent was left to the discretion of the researchers themselves. Until the Second World War medical researchers claimed a right to self-regulation in their medical practice. Critical issues like the definition of an experiment, or the form in which consent had to be obtained, were thus unregulated and left to personal and professional interpretation.

This situation led to tragic abuses involving human subjects volunteering in biomedical research. Perhaps the most recognizable case of abuse was the syphilis study conducted by the Public Health Service in Tuskegee, Alabama, where between 1930 and 1972 a group of 399 poor African American syphilis patients had their treatment withheld to allow white, middle-class doctors to study the "natural evolution" of the disease. The research, based on racist assumptions about biological differences between African Americans and whites, was intended to compare the effects of syphilis among Tuskegee patients with a nineteenth-century study of untreated syphilis patients in Norway. The Tuskegee study had no scientific value, and the experiment provided no therapeutic benefit for the patients who had to contend with the disease untreated even though Salvarsan—the accepted drug in the early 1930s—and then penicillin in the 1940s had been demonstrated to be effective. Worse, the patients believed that by volunteering to collaborate in the research they would get medical care. Over more than three uninterrupted decades the experiment involved a large number of researchers, research centers, and regulatory agencies. The study went through numerous reviews by the Public Health Service, which initiated it without major reservations, and the results were published in medical journals. Ultimately the story leaked to the press and the study was canceled amid much public indignation and criticism. During Bill Clinton's presidency the last survivors were offered an official apology. A judicial settlement had offered them financial compensation some years earlier.

Tuskegee is a tragic example of how racism, science, and state power interacted to shape biomedical research involving human subjects. It also illustrates the potential for ethical abuse of patients subjected to experimentation. But the abuses resulting from Tuskegee, shocking as they are, do not stand alone. The Second World War fueled a surge in research involving human subjects. Japan experimented with biological and chemical weapons in Manchuria, killing thousands of Chinese citizens; Germany subjected prisoners of war to depressurization chambers, tests of freezing effects, and exposure to chemical and biological agents. The United States also conducted war experiments. For example, because of concerns about infertility among those producing and manipulating atomic bombs, prisoners were exposed to radioactive materials to test its effects on male reproduction (Moreno 2000). This experiment was secret, its documentation was classified, and volunteers were not informed about the conditions of the trial in which they were involved.

Abuses during the war made evident the need to define a clear set of rules regarding human subjects' participation in biomedical research. In 1947 the Nuremberg Code established guidelines for the protection of human subjects in clinical trials, including a requirement that trial participants must make a voluntary declaration of consent, and a declaration of the patient's right to receive information on the nature, purpose, risks, and benefits of the experiments and to withdraw at any time. According to the code, the anticipated benefits of the trial must outweigh the risks. Some American scientists argued that this regulation applied to German scientists only and were not needed for their practice in the United States. As they had done in the pre-war period, medical professionals insisted on the benefits of self-regulation. For example, the director of the Public Health Service's division of venereal disease, which oversaw the Tuskegee experiment, saw no connection between experiments on Jewish prisoners in concentration camps and the research at Tuskegee (Jones 1993).

In 1974 the U.S. Congress passed the National Research Act, which established a National Commission for the Protection of Human Subjects of Biomedical and Behavioral Research. Its recommendations were issued in the Belmont Report in 1979. The report placed America in line with the spirit of the Nuremberg Code, on which the guidelines in the report were explicitly based. One of the central requirements was that scientists must receive proper training to conduct trials. However, the main contribution of the Belmont Report was its provision for independent institutional review boards (IRBS) to oversee the participation of human subjects. Board members, both professional and lay, had to guarantee the conditions regarding the informed-consent process. Volunteers needed to be fully informed of the risks and benefits of the trials. Recognizing that certain people could not be assumed to exercise free will, the Belmont Report placed limits on the participation in clinical trials of certain populations: children, the mentally ill, and institutionalized subjects like prisoners.

The shift from collegial, or professional, self-regulation to a more formalized, institutionalized regulation of human subjects' participation cannot be adequately explained as the product of the state's response to scandals and public outcry. A better explanation is that social movements during the 1960s against racial apartheid and in support of civil and human rights provided the context in which demands for ethical treatment of human subjects could be articulated and implemented.

The Belmont Report and subsequent laws resulted in new institutional arrangements to protect human subjects. IRBS and federal agencies such as the Office for the Protection of Research Subjects became part of the landscape. The Belmont Report's recommendation that prisoners be banned from clinical trials had a dramatic effect on the social organization of trials, forcing the pharmaceutical industry to devise strategies for finding new, suitable research subjects. In 1980, one year after the Belmont Report was issued, the Food and Drug Administration banned the participation of prisoners in clinical trials, since they were judged unable to give informed consent while subject to the institutional constraints of prison. This regulation signaled the end of the enrollment of institutionalized populations and the shift to a market approach. Until then prisoners had been the main source of paid human subjects for the pharmaceutical industry, and were the industry's preferred research subjects. An estimated 90 percent of drugs licensed before 1970 were first tested on prisoners (Harkness 1996). Prisoners were in many ways a perfect population for a controlled experiment. Because they had similar living conditions they provided good control groups for clinical trials, while the financial and material benefits ensured a large supply of willing and compliant volunteers.

Paid volunteers recruited through market mechanisms were more expensive and demanded new institutional arrangements. Publicity, recruiting centers, screening procedures, and selection guidelines were implemented to recruit a new population of paid subjects. As shown in chapter 1, the pharmaceutical industry's quest was not just for human volunteers but for an idealized body, healthy, disciplined, and willing. Over time the professionalization of subjects' participation ensured the pharmaceutical industry with the reliable research population it needed. However, the commodification of volunteers would not have been possible without another concomitant development: the emergence about the same time of the randomized clinical trial (RCT), which helped to shape the social organization of clinical-trials research.

RCT: THE GOLD STANDARD OF CLINICAL-TRIALS RESEARCH

Randomized clinical trials involving paid volunteers recruited on the open market and regulated by the state are a relatively new phenomenon. In 1962 the Kefauver-Harris Drug Amendment established the need to assess not only the safety of a drug—required by the FDA since 1938—but also its efficacy. In 1938 a drug commercially named Elixir Sulfanilamide containing a powerful, toxic ingredient (diethyl glycol) went on the market, causing 103 deaths before it was withdrawn. As a consequence the FDA demanded that the drug companies provide evidence regarding the safety of all drugs on the market. Until then the Pure Food and Drug Act of 1906 had only required that pharmaceutical companies label their products accurately and disclose the chemical composition of their formulas.

Kefauver-Harris, which added the requirement of "well controlled clinical investigations," contained no explicit mention of RCTs, but these soon became the standard for biomedical research, using statistical models that had already been introduced in agronomy and biology in the postwar era. "By 1970, short-term clinical trials were well established as a legal Standard of therapeutic efficacy and as a Standard of excellence in medical research. Although randomized trials were hardly universal in clinical medicine, they were far more common than they have been two decades earlier" (Marks 1997, 195).

According to Marks, the implementation of RCT demanded and was encouraged by new forms of specialization and scientific knowledge.

Statisticians view the RCT as the ideal experimental design, one that eliminated the bias of the observer in interpreting the outcome. An earlier generation's trust in the judgment of experienced researchers was to be replaced by reliance on an experimental method: "The use of properly designed clinical trials permits us to move from an authoritative frame of reference to a scientific one" (Marks 1997, 147).

Most medical researchers agreed. But not all medical doctors did. Having relied on personal experience with their patients as the basis for knowledge, many physicians had trouble accepting the idea of randomization and double-blind testing. Ultimately the disputes centered on the authority of statistics versus personal experience as a way of producing knowledge. Marks argues that despite these conflicts, the RCT was finally adopted because statisticians' emphasis on the need to raise the standards of therapeutic experimentation created a natural alliance with medical reformers who sought to improve the practice of medicine. In so doing, statisticians joined these reformers as part of a larger self-proclaimed progressive movement. Supporters of the progressive movement were mainly educated, middle-class Americans who believed that social reform was necessary and that the best way to achieve it was by employing scientific principles in an organized, modern, and systematic fashion. Reform of the American Medical Association, the creation of licensing organizations, stricter professional control, and the restructuring of medical education are typical reformist undertakings. Medical reformists in particular directed their efforts to regularizing and professionalizing medical practice through "modern" science and rationality. This group made a particular effort to distinguish between professionally trained physicians on the one hand and alternative practitioners and quacks on the other. The use of statistics was part of the rationalization and scientificity that they advocated for medicine, and the battle around its implementation in medical practice reflected conflicting professional and ideological views in a changing field.

If the adoption of RCTs was controversial among medical researchers, it presented still more problems for the pharmaceutical industry. The Kefauver-Harris act of 1962 did not mention RCTs, and the regulations implementing it were not enacted until 1970. Upjohn filed suit to challenge the act, alleging that the commercial success of a drug was substantial evidence of its safety and efficacy, but the court rebuffed the argument, holding that a drug's safety and efficacy should be proved by well-controlled clinical trials.

As discussed earlier, double-blind RCTs using placebos are now such a dominant model in clinical-trials research that eliminating the placebo requirement in tests of AIDS drugs took years of social mobilization by AIDS activists, who argued that using placebos on AIDS patients was unethical and was intended only to boost the industry's claims of drug efficacy. While it is impossible to ascertain what motivated the industry's response to the introduction of the RCT in the 1960s, there is no doubt that it has since come to embrace RCTs wholeheartedly.

THE QUEST FOR A "KNOWLEDGE ECONOMY" IN DEINDUSTRIALIZED PHILADELPHIA

In the decades following the Second World War Philadelphia experienced a process of deindustrialization. While this trend was also evident nationally and internationally, it was particularly strong in Philadelphia because of its manufacturing base, the extent of suburbanization in the region, and its dependence on unstable state and federal resources (Goode and Schneider 1994).

The city's industrial base relied heavily on the production of nondurable goods. In 1950 about 30 percent of Philadelphia's manufacturing jobs were in the nondurable sector, while the national average was 19 percent (Summers and Luce 1988). These industries were more sensitive to labor costs and had less fixed capital than producers of durable goods, and were thus less able to respond to changes in production technology and capital flows. As a result Philadelphia lost more of its manufacturing base than other large cities. One of the most severely affected sectors was textiles and apparel, which accounted for 25 percent of the city's total manufacturing employment in 1947. Between 1947 and 1986 this industry lost more than 97,000 jobs, an astonishing 74 percent of all jobs in the sector (Adams et al. 1991, 31). In total, Philadelphia lost nearly three-quarters of its manufacturing jobs between 1955 and 1990 (Stull and Madden 1990, 22; Adams et al. 1991, 30).

The extent of suburbanization aggravated the effects of deindustrialization in the city. Most of the city's population and jobs had relocated to the surrounding counties of the metropolitan region. While this pattern is by no means unique, data show that Philadelphia lost more economic activities to the suburbs than forty-two comparable standard metropolitan areas nationwide (Summers and Luce 1988). Between 1970 and 1980 the city lost 11.9 percent of its jobs, while there was an overall gain in the metropolitan area. For central cities nationwide, the average loss was 6.2 percent, which shows the greater impact of suburbanization in Philadelphia (Goode and Schneider 1994, 30).

Finally, the effects of deindustrialization on the city were increased by a declining tax base, coupled with a dramatic reduction in federal funds during the early 1980s.

Philadelphia struggled to reposition itself by relying heavily on the service economy, experiencing growth in finance, insurance, real estate, technology, legal services, and education. But other cities in the Northeast corridor such as New York, Washington, Boston, and Baltimore were doing the same thing (Goode and Schneider 1994, 31), and Philadelphia was ill prepared to match their economical and political advantages, especially in service industries like transportation and tourism. Goode shows that where Philadelphia had some success, as in its strategy of creating research and development parks focused on technology, like those in Boston and Raleigh-Durham, this has aided not the center city but the suburbs, especially in the Princeton corridor and along Route 202 near King of Prussia, a secondary central business district.

Despite setbacks, Philadelphia remains competitive in health care, higher education, and in particular biomedical and pharmaceutical research. The city is second only to New York as a location for medical schools, with more than twenty-five hospitals and ancillary institutions. Philadelphia also has two major universities. One of the most successful stories in the shift toward a service economy has been the city's ability to attract major pharmaceutical companies that work with the research departments of local universities. While there is some competition, especially from Baltimore and Boston, the city's tradition as a major pharmaceutical center gives it a competitive advantage in the pursuit of a knowledge economy. Currently major international drug companies like GlaxoSmithKline, Wyeth, Merck, and Bristol-Meyers Squibb have their headquarters or conduct clinical-trials research in the Philadelphia metropolitan area.

Philadelphia had been the center of the pharmaceutical industry in the country since the early nineteenth century, when the first local chemical manufacturers were established. Until 1812 America had imported its medicines from Britain, but the war disrupted this trade and created opportunities for local apothecaries. According to Liebenau, many pharmacies could expand into laboratories to begin large-scale production with relative ease, since the industry has low capital requirements and only a general knowledge of pharmaceutical practice was required. The simplicity of the procedures also allowed considerable diversification, which facilitated the development of wide markets and the strategic use of particular product lines according to demand (Liebenau 1987, 12). Foreign-trained pharmacists founded many of the new companies in the second decade of the nineteenth century, and these firms came to dominate the American chemical and pharmaceutical industry into the twentieth century. A good representative was Smith, Kline and French, which had acquired its apothecary license in 1829 and by the middle of the century was already well established. Around this time Philadelphia and New York became the main suppliers of drugs—mainly imported from London—that they distributed through marketing networks to satisfy urban and rural demand.

The Civil War represented a huge opportunity for the industry in Philadelphia, which according to the census of manufacturers showed significant growth between 1860 and 1870. According to Liebenau the number of establishments manufacturing medicines, extracts, and drugs rose from 173 to 292, and the number employed in them more than quadrupled, from 1,059 to 4,729, while capital investment grew even more, from $1,977,385 to $12,750,809. After the war, Powers and Weightman, Rosengarten and Sons, Smith Kline, Wyeth, and smaller manufacturers all expanded. By the 1870s medical manufacturers in Philadelphia dominated the region and supplied the bulk of the southern and western markets, aided by developments in communications and transportation. Able to exploit national markets by 1890, many drug companies grew substantially, displacing less successful competitors. In Philadelphia Smith Kline grew to the detriment of Wyeth and other businesses to become the city's most important dealer. Other regional players also gained considerable local and national muscle. Squibb and Merck in New York and Parke Davis, Lilly, and Upjohn also extended their markets.

As some companies grew their laboratories began to employ scientists emerging from medical schools who had acquired scientific knowledge about bacteriological and biochemical processes. Philadelphia's position as an outstanding medical center played an important role in bringing medical science to the attention of the pharmaceutical industry. However, the companies did not start immediately to produce drugs based on scientific principles, instead assuming "more of the veneer than the substance of scientific medicine" (Liebeneau 1987, 41) Usually the pharmaceutical industry's claims to science did not led to the installation of science-based laboratories. Despite the industry's scientific pretensions, the labs did not resemble the research centers of their counterparts in Germany.

From the beginning the pharmaceutical industry in the United States was a mixture of science and big business (Balis 2000). In Germany its development was based on different premises. Organic chemistry began in the 1860s, when the molecular structure of basic carbon compounds was deciphered. In the second half of the nineteenth century Germany expanded and improved its training of chemists. It was these scientists who founded an organic chemistry industry. Their research into coal-tar products led after 1880 to a synthetic drug industry. Aspirin was among the first and most successful of German pharmaceutical products. From similar research lines came Paul Ehrlich's development of Salvarsan, an efficacious drug for treating syphilis. The German industry retained its connection to its scientific roots and was controlled by a technically trained directorate until the second decade of the twentieth century. The link between academic training and industry remained strong. Germany dominated the international chemical market and was almost the exclusive worldwide producer of coal-tar-based dyes and other drugs until the First World War.

By contrast, the United States had relatively unsophisticated technological origins and lacked a strong connection between the academic training of chemists and the new chemical industry. (For a more complete description of the relationship between academic and industrial pharmacology see Swann 1984.) For many firms the use of science meant merely an effort to increase drug standardization. Two directories were published to inform doctors about drugs. One was the United States Pharmacopoeia, published every ten years, listing drugs and preparations. The other was the National Formulary, which contained pharmaceutical formulas in current use.

In the course of their efforts to reform medicine, the American Medical Association established the Council on Pharmacy and Chemistry in 1905. The purpose of the council was to encourage doctors to move against the forces that resisted the advancement of "rational therapy." It was also intended to discourage the use of patented drugs by physicians. The council provided the standards that would allow physicians to prescribe ethical drugs with confidence. It was also an attempt on the part of the AMA to gain some degree of disciplinary control over the pharmaceutical industry. In 1906 the AMA established its own chemical laboratory with the cooperation of the American Pharmaceutical Association. It published its own definitions of acceptable drugs, as well as appropriate drug analysis and standards. Only those drugs that had been accepted for inclusion could be advertised in professional medical journals. With the passage of the pure Food and Drug Act of 1906 the standards of the Pharmacopoeia and the National Formulary took on the force of law.

According to Liebenau, standardization, the employment of scientists, and even a small laboratory did not necessarily imply a significant shift in a company's outlook during the last decades of the nineteenth century (Liebenau 1987, 46). He argues that even as the pharmaceutical industry used science as a promotional and marketing device, scientific knowledge was not incorporated into the drug development process. Yet Liebenau acknowledges that by the first decade of the twentieth century many American pharmaceutical companies had adopted science not only at the rhetorical level but also in their production lines. Many of their products emerged from the laboratories, and the companies emphasized their scientific qualities; science was now used to define whether a company had attained standards of quality (Liebenau 1987, 79). Science-based laboratories helped to increase drug standardization, which appealed to physicians, giving the companies a competitive advantage. Also, the use of science in pharmaceutical laboratories helped the industry to differentiate its products from "quack" proprietary drugs, enhancing the modern, scientific image of pharmaceutical companies.

The Pure Food and Drug Act regulating drug production had demanded truth in labeling. To comply with the law each drug had to be accurately assayed and labeled as to its contents. This requirement made the equipment of laboratories a necessary expense for all ethical drug companies, which accepted the necessity of doing so as a way to distinguish themselves from the manufacturers of patent medicines. Drugs were divided into two categories, proprietary and ethical. Proprietary drugs were patented substances. Their formulas were kept secret and they were advertised to the general public. Ethical drugs were advertised only to the medical profession and their ingredients and patent information were disclosed. Only patented medicines were prepackaged. For ethical drugs, the pharmacist or physician prepared the prescription. There were, however, no stipulations attached to the prescription. The druggist could make up enough for a whole family or package and sell the doctor's prescription to the general public (unless the drug contained opium).

The Pure Food and Drug Act of 1906 was a response to the demand that state regulation be standardized, along with pressure from such large pharmaceutical manufacturers as Smith Kline and French. The companies wished to exploit their near-monopoly on certain markets and the facilities of their laboratories, and to reduce competition by driving out smaller producers (Liebenau 1987). Liebenau argues that the Pure Food and Drug Act rationalized the industry, forcing out of business small producers, mainly proprietary drug producers, who could not afford to equip themselves properly. The large pharmaceutical industries insisted on a high standard of purity. As a result of the legislation the number of companies competing in the marketplace declined while large companies with analytical laboratories continued to thrive.

An alliance between ethical drug firms and medicine was being forged in the name of science, and in opposition to proprietary medicines. The analytical laboratory was already well equipped by the turn of the century. The labs performed two functions: protecting the company from the purchase of inferior raw materials and standardizing its finished products.

The pharmaceutical industry thus advanced with the aid of technological advancements, scientific ambitions, and governmental regulations. The First World War provided a political incentive for the United States government to suspend German patents, allowing American companies to further accumulate capital by producing previously German-patented drugs. We witness here the complex interactions among capital development, government regulation, science, and medicine. With the beginning of the First World War supplies from Germany became unreliable, further inducing America to produce its own chemicals and medicinals. While drug producers used patriotic rhetoric to abrogate German patents, thus using German technology to develop an American chemical industry (Balis 2000), only large companies benefited from this development, since the industry had become technically sophisticated, requiring considerable equipment and investments in fixed capital.

The pharmaceutical industry emerged from the First World War stronger than before. Large government contracts and the acquisition of patents provided the bases for growth. Helped by significant resources thanks to the acquisition of German patents in the 1920s, drug companies began to build solid research facilities. G. D. Searle opened a lab in 1924, followed by Smith Kline and French in 1925 and Burroughs Wellcome (USA) in 1928. Other companies with minimal research staffs expanded them in the late 1920s and 1930s. The Institute for Therapeutic Research was opened by Merck in 1933, a research laboratory by Eli Lilly in 1934, the Institute for Medical Research by Squibb in 1938, and the Abbott Research Lab also in 1938 (Swann 1995, 81). Industrial applications of organic chemistry in the United States became important only after bureaucratic and industrial structures had developed, and after a class of industrial management appeared (Balis 2000, 34). Mergers and takeovers within the chemical industry in the 1920s led to stronger managerial structures as well as scientific expansion. (Liebenau 1987). The business of pharmaceuticals evolved within the context of the changing nature of American capitalism, but it was also shaped by the rapid development of pharmacology, which emerged as an important academic discipline during the end of the nineteenth century and the beginning of the twentieth. Furthermore, the relationship between academic and industrial pharmacology changed significantly in the interwar years, and this had a profound effect on the shape of the emerging drug business.

For many drug companies the rhetoric of science was an important way of redefining, repositioning, and legitimizing themselves. This reflected a change in marketing strategy as well as changes in the product. In this context, it is perhaps understandable that academic pharmacologists in the United States should have distanced themselves from the pharmaceutical industry, fearing commercial exploitation. Over time, the need for funding, combined with assiduous courtship from the industry, broke their resistance (Swann 1988).

After the Second World War the industry experienced a period of growth and also of specialization along particular product lines. Large producers that before the war had offered thousands of products centered their efforts on just a few. Small businesses that wanted to thrive had a strong incentive to merge with larger companies if they wanted to keep producing ethical drugs. Although the demands during the war for penicillin and antibiotics had sped up the organization of the pharmaceutical business, furthering research and product development on an unprecedented scale, Liebenau argues that the new structures, involving marketing as well as research, and the industry's relationship with academic scientists and medical doctors had been built much earlier, during the years preceding the Great Depression (Liebenau 1987, 134).

THE SERVICE ECONOMY AND THE EMERGENCE OF
THE PROFESSIONAL RESEARCH SUBJECT

The shift toward a service economy in Philadelphia had—as in many other large urban areas—dramatic effects not only at the top of the social scale but also at the bottom. If for well-educated, entrepreneurial professionals the new economy provided new opportunities, the same was not true of occupations at the lower level. The shift to the service sector, in which 75 percent of the workforce in metropolitan Philadelphia is now employed, did not fully make up for manufacturing job losses. Moreover, the service economy provides employment with few or no health or retirement benefits, and lower wages. At the same time it produces a deskilling of the workforce, making the industrial apprenticeship something of the past. As a result, workers in the service economy move from one job to the next without acquiring any new skills that can lead to their upward mobility.

One of the most distressing effects of the shift from an industrial to a service economy in Philadelphia has been the emergence of a mass of vulnerable, unemployed, or poorly employed workers. This group, along with others from around the country, contributes to fill the slots in the emergent clinical-trials industry. This process has been documented abroad by Rajan, who describes how unemployed workers in the trials economy in India are subjected to speculative regimes of scientific research and capital accumulation. "Just so, in Mumbai, one can see how forced deproletarization, as a consequence of a shift in modes of production from manufacturing to commercial capitalism, leads to the virtual death of an entire industry and to the creation of a new population of subjects who are retrenched workers and subjects of experimental therapeutic intervention" (Rajan 2005, 26).

7

ETHICS AND THE EXPLOITATION OF
THE POOR IN CLINICAL TRIALS RESEARCH

TRANSLATING RISK

The informed-consent form is the most important source of information about phase I of a clinical trial. It details the design, purpose, procedures, risks, and benefits for human subjects. As mentioned in chapter 3, volunteers perceive themselves as well informed or very well informed about the risks involved in the trials they have joined. A review of a semi-structured survey that I conducted among eighteen professional guinea pigs confirms this perception. Of those who had volunteered in the preceding six months to a year, two-thirds of respondents remembered the sponsor of the trial, the drug or drugs being tested, and the goal and main risks mentioned in the informed-consent form.

During my fieldwork I also had the opportunity to follow numerous professional guinea pigs volunteering in diverse settings. I questioned them after they had received the informed-consent form upon qualifying for the trial and again after they signed it upon enrollment. Michael, whose case was introduced in chapter 1, offers a good example of the way volunteers understand and respond to the informed-consent form. He was first exposed to the form once he was selected to enter the trial. At this point he had an interview with a registered nurse who explained to him the basic components of the trial. A few days later he entered the trial at Jefferson and on his first day he, along with the other volunteers, had the opportunity to ask questions about the informed-consent form before signing it. I met him after he had received the form, and he told me he had trouble getting through it. It was thick, he said. He had asked no questions to the nurse who had handed it to him. He knew who the sponsor was, but could not tell what was the purpose of the study. And while he recognized that the trial was a controlled randomized trial (CTR)—like most trials—he was confused about the complex design, involving different drug dosages and control groups. While reviewing the form he noticed that the drug had been tested before on dogs and rats. While nothing happened with rats, one dog had died. I asked him about this. Was he concerned? No, he wasn't, he told me. He was just pointing out the fact to me, he said, not knowing what to make of it. It was a much larger dose than the one he would get, he said. Finally, Michael could not describe the schedule, which consisted of a number of days as an inpatient, a wash-out period, and then another period as an inpatient. What Michael remembered very well was that the study was a two-week, inpatient study at Jefferson and that he would pocket $2,700 at completion.

After Michael had his first break from the trial I met him again, and we talked about the trial's informed-consent form. This was just two weeks after he first received the form and a few days after he had entered the trial, and this time Michael had a much better idea of the trial goals, design, and risks. In response to my question, he said that he understood the trial better as it progressed. As we have seen in chapter 3, the interaction with other professional guinea pigs before and during the trial plays a crucial role in shaping volunteers' understanding of the trial's design, schedule, organization, and risks.

Also, time is important in shaping volunteers' understanding of a trial. Michael's knowledge increased over time. When he was first handed the informed-consent after being accepted but before volunteering, he understood very little. After signing and volunteering, he understood more. By the end of the trial he was able to recite every minor detail concerning the goal of the trial, the drug being tested, the schedule, and the risks.

During the trial the informed-consent form had also changed. After the trial started Michael was handed another copy of the form announcing some changes to the protocol. Fifteen new members had been added to the study, and the sponsor was legally required to inform volunteers of any modifications. Michael was not concerned by this change. However, another change did affect him. He was to receive a $700 bonus for his trial participation. He told me he was happy about the money, but he also wondered why it was being given to him. Was there something risky or nasty about the trial? Not that he was very worried. "Easy money," he told me.

The informed-consent form elicits a number of responses, associations, anxieties, and demands among professional guinea pigs. Some of their anxieties are the product of incomplete or misleading information about the design and risks associated with the trial. One source of concern, as we have seen with Michael, is changes introduced to the informed-consent form once a trial has started. The Canadian guinea pig with a few trials behind him in the United States perceived himself as being very well informed about the risks he might face, but changes in the form also give him pause. I asked him how well informed he was about the risks and benefits of the trials. "Usually very informed. Sometimes the form is not very clear. Most of the time it is because they write procedures out and then they add things later at the last minute, and they change the informed consent. Sometimes it happens when the study is about to start and sometimes it happens when the study has already started and that pisses a lot of people off" (Canadian guinea pig, 4 July 2004).

Another source of concern for professional guinea pigs is the elusive scientific jargon embedded in the form. "They have to tell you everything that ever happened, but they say, for example: a large percentage of this population. They tell anything that ever happened when the drug was tested and then they say this stuff probably won't happen to you. A lot of people have this problem with the informed consent. I think that my fear in relation to risk is not so much what they know and are not telling you. It's what they don't know" (Spam, 28 July 2004).

Spam's concern is not that scientists might withhold information about risks but that the uncertainties of research make risk assessment uncertain. One of the main unknowns of phase I studies, as mentioned in chapter 1, is the difficulty of extrapolating toxicological results from animals to humans. That a substance has been shown to be nontoxic for animals does not mean that it is nontoxic for humans, which is precisely what the phase I trial is designed to prove. These kinds of risks are embedded in the structural design of the trials. This element disturbed Spam and other guinea pigs. Commenting on this issue, Dave Onion told me: "I know what it does in rats," implying that he did not know its effects on human beings.

Professional guinea pigs' responses to the informed-consent process reflect their uneasiness about being paid to participate in clinical-trials research. As I have shown in earlier chapters, it is not scientific advancement or altruism that motivates them to volunteer. With no illusions about the pharmaceutical industry's intentions in drug research, volunteers only engage in the trial economy for financial gain. They are well aware of the commodification of their bodies and, as we have seen, resent the dehumanizing treatment they receive as research subjects. While they define themselves as workers in a contractual relationship, they also see that the relationship has exploitative, coercive elements and as Frank Little illustrates, the informed-consent form is seen in that light.

> I was saying it's a fundamentally coercive relationship but any time money is being exchanged for a service—even if this service is consensual—the person needs the money to survive, I mean, it's a coercive relationship, there's no way around it. So, because of that, you know, it's a coercive relationship so, I am consenting to participate, I am not being forced to but I need the money and I know that and they know that. It's a business relationship. It's a contractual relationship, I am not certainly doing it out of the goodness of my heart and they are not paying me out of the goodness of their heart, they are paying me because they know this is the only way they are going to get people to do the studies. There are not a lot of people that are out there that want to put experimental medication in their body for the hell of it. So, I think that the big thing they are paying people for is, because there is a lot of people that are out there and this is an easy way to make money taking experimental medication. So, the pharmaceutical companies that are doing this, they are exploiting that, they are exploiting the need that people have for money. (Frank Little, 12 September 2004)

COMMODIFICATION AND ETHICS IN TRIALS RESEARCH
AMONG PROFESSIONAL GUINEA PIGS

I have argued that the pharmaceutical industry denies the commodification of the body in clinical-trials research by employing a number of semantic turns that mask the identity of their subjects. Thus professional research subjects become "paid volunteers" compensated for their "time and efforts." Similarly, informed-consent forms contain hypertechnical language and avoid references to risks, suffering, and death. Scott, a close friend and collaborator of Helms who has been doing clinical trials in Philadelphia for more than ten years, explains his anxiety over this point:

You have to go to [doctors and staff] with demands. I am not saying you should do it in a confrontational way, but you have to go with the mindset that these people are over here and you are down here, you have to make sure that your communication is appropriate for that kind of relationship. It doesn't mean that you are going to scream at them but you go and say: "OK, I am not going to do the study until you explain what an anaphylactic reaction is." This is an example for a study I did once. They were reading down the informed consent and they were going, like, this is a phase 1 study. First time in man, we did it with animals already and she is saying that the dose, twenty times over the normal rate, would produce an anaphylactic reaction in 60 percent of the animals. And I was like: "What is an anaphylactic reaction?" She paused, "Well, it's when your heart stops beating and your lungs stop breathing." Then I said: "That means that you are dead?" and she replied: "As long as it doesn't start again, yes." That's good to know. (Scott, 3 June 2004)

By challenging the wording of informed-consent forms, demanding less technical and more understandable language to refer to procedures and risks, and reclaiming the dignity and value of the work they do as professional guinea pigs, volunteers bring commodification to the forefront of phase I clinical-trials research. Their recognition of the commodification of their bodies prompts them to challenge the ethics of clinical-trials research under the current institutional arrangements. As I showed in chapter 2, *Guinea Pig Zero* attempted to provide a narrative of the history and present circumstances of human subjects in biomedical research, from the point of view of human guinea pigs and in defense of their interests. One of its key issues was advocacy of an ethical standard that reflected volunteers' concerns instead of those of industrial, professional, or institutional groups. Helms, the editor, covered a number of historical cases of abuse involving human subjects. He also paid attention to the informed-consent process, making it one of the most important criteria used in the writing of report cards of research sites. Helms noted that laws and regulations cannot adequately protect volunteers. Affirming his anarchist identity, which was shared by most of the professional guinea pigs in West Philadelphia, Helms relied not on institutions but on the possibilities of individual and collective organized action: "The courts are not going to protect you, the government is not going to protect you. Take advantage of the numbers, take advantage of getting together when the management does not expect you to get together, be very careful, avoid situations like serotonin drug trials, avoid psychiatrists like the plague. In other words, the authorities, the regulators, the courts, they are not there to protect you if you are working class or a guinea pig, anybody in the low end of the totem pole. Your brains, your strategy, and your getting together, and above all, never believing in them, never believing in authorities, you believe in yourself and what it is real about yourself" (Helms, 15 January 2005).

Despite the ideological cohesion among the anarchist and other radical volunteers, some members have slightly different views of the role of legal and regulatory bodies in safeguarding the well-being and ethical treatment of human subjects in research. While all had the same identity as guinea pigs and similar experiences and views of commodification in phase I research, some members expressed a pragmatic conviction that institutions could play a positive role in protecting them. "Of course that in a lot of levels I don't trust them. In the bottom line they are making the money. But at the same time, because their bottom line is making the money, at a certain level I don't think they are going to be honest with me out of the goodness of their hearts but I think that they are going to be honest with me because they want to protect their backs. So in this sense I trust that the information they give me about secondary effects and so forth is very accurate because they don't want to be hit with a big lawsuit. So, in this sense, I trust them but it's not, as I said, because these are altruistic companies that are out there to do good, it's because they want to protect their own interests, which is not to be hit with a big lawsuit" (Frank Little, 12 September 2004).

Shon, another volunteer, expressed the same conviction about the positive effects of state regulation: "I think that there is an interesting question you raised about state regulation. While I was working in truck driving in California I noticed that the regulation on truck driving was much more lax than other kinds of driving regulations so I wanted to do something about it in that context of deaths on the job and also as an "anti" status. The thing is that biomedical research is much more regulated and I am happy that it is regulated to the degree it is now, especially compared to the research previously done on prisoners, the Tuskegee experiment. Compared to that history I am very happy for the state intervention on that. I can also imagine a society where the regulation would be done by the social and not by the state, through the participation of interested citizens and independent boards" (Shon, 2 June 2004).

Frank's and Shon's views of governmental regulation are not totally at odds with their radical beliefs. Perhaps their positions should be viewed as only tactically different, though born of a common recognition that sometimes the system is able to guard against the worst abuses in research. As Shon also recognizes, ethical protections for human subjects have evolved in the last decades, rising to a level not afforded to previous generations.

INFORMED CONSENT AMONG HIV VOLUNTEERS

Like the professional guinea pigs, HIV patients volunteering at CBTO relied on the informed-consent form as a means of acquiring information about trial designs, goals, risks, and benefits. In addition, patients at CBTO consulted with their personal doctors and the staff in charge of their trials before making a decision. This reflects an important difference between the two groups. As we have seen, while professional guinea pigs do not trust the scientists or the pharmaceutical industry, CBTO volunteers have a trusting relationship with their doctors and researchers. However, a small group of African American volunteers at CBTO had concerns about the ethics of trials and mentioned past abuses involving African Americans, in particular at Tuskegee. These patients trust their doctors but also feel that the doctors are not disclosing everything about risks. They expressed their belief that if researchers were completely forthcoming, volunteers would not volunteer.

When I began my fieldwork at CBTO in the spring of 2004, all the volunteers had been enrolled in their trials, some for years. Unfortunately, this prevented me from observing how they understood the informed-consent form at the moment of signing. As a result, I could not do the same kind of follow-up that I had done with professional guinea pigs who volunteered for phase I trials. However, data from a survey that I administered to this population shed some light on their knowledge of the trial they were in and its goals, design, risks, and benefits.

The majority of twenty patients interviewed at CBTO declared that they saw themselves as being well informed or very well informed about the risks they faced when they became volunteers. Most patients were able to correctly identify the trial they were in, its goals, the drug or drugs involved (if any), and the main risks and benefits. Some patients had trouble identifying the sponsor of the trial. Instead of naming the institution that supported the study, they would name their doctor at CBTO, or the principal investigator of the study, or more frequently the staff member they regularly saw when making a visit in connection with the study. This confusion had no practical consequences and might have reflected the complex social organization of trials at CBTO, where "industry" trials were held together with "community" trials.

This high level of understanding is not surprising, given that HIV patients, as we saw in chapter 5, engage in the trials as part of their strategy of coping with their disease. Trials are an opportunity to get access to drugs and better health care, and to help advance efforts to understand and treat the virus. As mentioned in chapter 6, many volunteers have experience in community organizations, experience that has made them empowered "consumers" who play an active role in their health care. Some, for instance, have completed community-based educational programs, at CBTO and elsewhere, on the ethics of biomedical research in HIV trials.

It is not possible to compare the effects of financial compensation on informed-consent processes among phase I professional guinea pigs and HIV trial volunteers. As mentioned, all HIV trial volunteers were enrolled in trials when interviewed, while some professional guinea pigs had undergone trials months or even years earlier. The difference in time shaped the way the participants remembered their trial experiences and their recollections regarding the informed-consent process. Furthermore, differences in trial design exist not only between the groups but among HIV volunteers at CBTO. While a trial such as SMART tested the effects of a controlled interruption of drug treatment, others such as the Tipranavir-Norvir trial tested the efficacy of combining different drugs.

The wide differences in financial compensation also explains the contrasting attitudes toward the ethics of trials research and the informed-consent process. Professional guinea pigs are very critical of the informed-consent process and existing oversight of ethics. In contrast, apart from those who had some anxiety over past research abuses, HIV volunteers were generally unconcerned. They trust their doctors and institutions, and hope that clinical trials will benefit them, or help scientific advance-ment, or both. As we saw in chapter 6, financial compensation played a role in motivating one-third of the patients in HIV trials, but it was not the main impetus, nor did it shape their identity or their attitude toward the trials.

MONEY AND ETHICS AT CBTO

As noted in chapter 6, the local IRB oversees patients' rights, making sure that the informed-consent process is followed. First, the IRB decides whether a proposed trial involving HIV patients can be conducted. Once a trial is approved, the IRB has to ensure that informed consent is secured from the volunteers before they join the trial. I now explore how the local IRB approaches the informed-consent process and how its dealings with powerful pharmaceutical industry interests creates potential conflicts of interest.

The IRB places a high value on research, but some members are suspi-cious of the pharmaceutical industry's motives for conducting HIV trials. "I haven't been involved with any regulatory bodies before, but I have a big belief in the value of research. And while I may be always skeptical of the motives of the pharmaceutical companies, and I am concerned about pharmaceutical companies making an inappropriate amount of money while rationing out an important product. I do think that research is fundamentally important in contributing to make a dent into the epi-demic" (IRB's chair, 17 August 2004). The IRB chair's endorsement of research echoes that of CBTO; this commitment to research has been characteristic of the organization since its founding by a group of HIV doctors and activists who believed that without community involvement in research, progress would be slow. On the other hand, the IRB chair is a community AIDS lawyer and activist, and his concern with the profit-driven pharmaceutical industry recalls the denunciation by AIDS organiza-tions of market-driven HIV research that makes access to promising drugs difficult for poor patients at home and abroad.

CBTO's principal investigator and liaison with the pharmaceutical in-dustry trials, while strongly endorsing the pharmaceutical industry con-tributions, also has a more nuanced view of this relationship. He initially seems to fully endorse the role of the pharmaceutical industry in the fight against HIV:

Clearly, in HIV the patient's interest is the heart here, and what we really care for is our patients in a sense. As you know, HIV advancement has been industry driven. All of the advances made in HIV have been made thanks to the efforts of the pharmaceutical industry. All the drugs that have been manufactured for HIV that are life-saving are not manufactured by NIH or federal organizations. All the tests, resistance testing, viral load test, were manufactured by industry companies. So unfortunately we are obliged to collaborate with industry, because they are the main players in this field. And if we want to be an entity involved in cutting-edge research there's no escape but to collaborate with the industry and that's what's happening. Unlike the CDC and vaccines, for example, or epidemiological studies where the CDC is very strong and you would want to collaborate with the government, in HIV if you don't have a good relationship in collaborating with industry companies you're nobody.

The people doing clinical trials for the industry are researchers, and we deal with the scientific part more than with the marketing part. When we do the trials we are not collaborating with the marketing people. We are dealing with the scientific liaison in the pharmaceutical company and the scientists are scientists, wherever they are they are scientists. They are very objective, they are very decent—their integrity is unquestionable—and we don't deal with marketing, we don't have anything to do with marketing. It's mainly the scientific committee of the company we are dealing with. (PI, 27 April 2004)

I could sense the principal investigator's excitement for recent developments in pharmaceutical research involving HIV drugs. As a doctor —very well respected and loved by his patients—he believed that new drugs offered him the possibility of improving the therapeutic chances of his patients, making them live longer or improving their quality of life. As a researcher, he was clearly inspired by the scientific advancements. He enthusiastically told me that "all the HIV drugs that are life-saving have been developed by the pharmaceutical industry. The CDC or the NIH had not made a significant contribution." He perceives scientists working for the pharmaceutical industry as being objective, their integrity unquestionable. The PI's rhetoric is strongly influenced by scientific discourses that stress the value of neutrality, objectivity, and progress. However, HIV community activists have challenged this view, arguing that science, ideology, and politics play a significant role in HIV drugs research. In particular, community advocates have denounced the contributions that the federal government has made in basic research through the CDC and the NIH, contributions that have led to breakthroughs later appropriated by the pharmaceutical industry. In this view, the public sector heavily subsidized the pharmaceutical industry by funding expensive and basic research that was the basis of drug development by the private sector. HIV community movements have also denounced racial, class, and gender biases in clinical-trials research for HIV drugs conducted by the industry, as well as what it considered the unethical use of placebos in HIV clinical trials, which withheld available therapies from patients in need of them.

This activist movement forced the industry to change the design of its HIV trials in the mid-1990s by testing an experimental drug against an existing HIV therapy instead of against a placebo. Social pressure from HIV advocates also forced the industry and the government to acknowledge that HIV trials needed to incorporate more African Americans and women into HIV research to reflect the spread of the epidemic.

Despite the principal investigator's support of the pharmaceutical research he is not willing to give the industry a blank check. Like the IRB chair, he recognizes that "unfortunately we are obliged to collaborate with industry companies because they are the main players in this field." Strategically, he sees the industry as being at the forefront of "cutting-edge" research from which CBTO can benefit. Like the community advocates, the PI is concerned that industry trials are frequently designed to maximize commercial claims instead of producing new knowledge:

RA: My question was focusing on the following. On one study you have Tipranavir and another drug, Norvir. Are they from the same company?

PI: No, Tipranavir is from [Boer Ingenham] and Norvir is from Abbott. It is not necessary that the two drugs belong to the same company. In the majority of the trials they do not, except in regime trials. Comparing two regimens among themselves, usually the drugs that you are comparing in the regime tend to come from the company that designs the trial. So the trial tries to use as many drugs as possible in this trial that are manufactured by the company. Most of the drugs are like these. For example, we are doing a trial for GSK comparing Kaletra to Lexiva. The backbone is Abacavir and 3TC, which are two drugs manufactured by GSK, it is not Tipranavir and 3TC, which is manufactured by another company. So the company that designs the trial tends to pick up the backbone based on the drug that the company manufactures.

That's the whole idea, to compare a drug against a preferred regimen to see if it does well or not. But the backbone, meaning the other two drugs in the regimen—usually comparing two drugs involve the same drugs in both arms—might not be the best option for the patient. If you had a chance to design the trial sometimes you wonder if that's the best thing for the patient, now that we know what's preferred and what's alternative. But again, it's always learning. Every time you are doing a trial you are learning more things about the combinations.

As we can see, researchers and IRB members alike are ambivalent about industry trials. They recognize the benefits that can derive from a relationship with the industry, but at the same time they fear that prospective financial gains can influence the research. These anxieties are reflected particularly in their views of the informed-consent process. Decisions such as those concerning which trials should be accepted and which should not show some of the tensions between the desire for scientific and therapeutic advancement and the protection of volunteers.

The local IRB is also concerned about the effects of increased body commodification brought about by financial incentives to recruit patients for trials. Although minimal at CBTO, the increasing presence of material rewards is perceived as an "undue influence" and a potential threat to the integrity of informed-consent process, in which volunteers are supposed to be able to evaluate risks and benefits independently of other considerations. "Well, I am always concerned about the influence that pharmaceutical companies can buy because they have a lot of money. The idea of patient compensation is a tricky one because why are you giving a patient twenty dollars if you stand to make millions. On the other hand, I want participants to balance risks and benefits by themselves, I don't want to see that balance unduly influenced by money. My concern is that if you offer me a lot of money instead of a little bit of money I might be more willing to overlook the risks and I am very concerned about that. I don't want to see participants overlook the risks, it should be a fully informed consent" (IRB chair, 17 August 2004).

Risk and benefit analysis is the standard way for prospective volunteers and IRBs to evaluate the merits of a trial involving human subjects. This criterion, first established in the Nuremberg Code in 1948, has since been widely adopted. Benefits anticipated from a trial should outweigh the risks to volunteers. CBTO's IRB considers the relationship between risk and benefits as the basis for any decision about trials, but first it considers whether the research question has any validity:

> We think about it in terms of analysis: first, we assess if there is a valid scientific question. Then we go on to the analysis of the risk and benefits of the study. Just to digress with that, if you look at Tuskegee, was that a valid scientific question? Well, I don't know if the question itself was invalid but then when you go to the risks and benefits, then we are off the table. So I think that is always the question of whether the research question is valid. If you look at the experiments during World War II, were they asking valid questions? The research was all over the place and there were no controls, maybe there was not even a valid question. I think that Tuskegee gives us a lot to think about in terms of interesting questions, maybe, maybe not.
>
> But the point is that once that you start getting to the risks and benefits analysis then it becomes an absolute no-no. (IRB's chair, 17 August 2004)

Needless to say, there was no science behind Tuskegee. However, the chair's point illustrates how the IRB approaches the issue. If the research question has no validity then the analysis of risks and benefits becomes irrelevant, and it becomes unethical to expose human subjects to prove a meaningless point. Deciding whether a question has scientific value presents problems for a body that is composed of professional and lay members.

> **RA:** I went to one IRB meeting and was surprised by the quality of the discussion, everybody was so engaged. You are a lawyer: how do you evaluate scientific claims?
>
> **IRB CHAIR:** It is very difficult. We are fortunate to have very knowledgeable doctors and very knowledgeable consumer representation. Because I am obviously not a medical person my role is to break things down even more basically. So, explain it to me very clearly, what would

they show? How would it help, and in the primary analysis if the help is for the pharmaceutical companies and not the patients then there is something that we are unlikely to approve.

In assessing the validity of the question one major consideration for the IRB is that the trial should be designed to answer a scientific question and not to produce a marketing claim for the pharmaceutical industry. Thus, every research protocol submitted for IRB approval is analyzed and scrutinized, having in mind the industry's desire to market the drug.

Some [were] too risky but most protocols we have rejected are similar to one we had just reviewed. The idea is this: we are looking at the question that is being asked. Is this a valid question, or is this a question that is really designed to give the pharmaceutical companies better marketing?—Well, not marketing but better claims about their drugs. Is the trial structured in such a way that the results can only give favorable results? Geez! Taking two of our drugs in combination is better than taking only one of our drugs. So, now they can sell two of their drugs. We are concerned when we see protocols that are more designed to enhance the reputation of the drug, a particular company, rather than to benefit the participant. (IRB's chair, 17 August 2004)

While the IRB has rejected numerous "industry" trials in recent years because they failed to prove scientific or therapeutic merit, the question of whether a drug trial has scientific merit or is driven by marketing claims does not provide a clear-cut answer. When the PI receives a study from the pharmaceutical companies that he feels is not suitable to be conducted at CBTO, he does not return it to the company. Instead he sends it to the IRB and in this way can kill the project without losing face with the pharmaceutical industry. "Yes, we bring the protocol to the IRB meeting. It is a fair way. When you want to kill a project we are successful doing it at the IRB meeting. But sometimes I wanted to carry a project and the IRB killed it. It happened to me. And I tell you; the IRB perceives new drugs as high-risk studies. And this was a new drug and they wanted [the pharmaceutical industry], you know, to start looking to the safety profile of this drug and trying to determine the right dosing, so this was like a phase II and the IRB didn't like the idea. They didn't like the idea that the pharmaceutical company wanted to know about the pharmacokinetics of the drug and this was shut down by the IRB" (PI, 27 April 2004).

According to its PI, the IRB at CBTO is so jealous in safeguarding the well-being of its patients that sometimes it kills trials that the PI thought had merit. Drug safety trials present no therapeutic benefit and represent a concern for the IRB. Most of the trials conducted at CBTO are of drugs that are in the latest stages of development or are already in the market but are being tested for a different application.

What seems unusual in the workings of this local IRB is that unlike others that had been criticized for following a formalistic, legalistic approach to informed consent, members at CBTO engage in a discussion that goes beyond the formal issues. As the IRB chair's remarks illustrate, lay and professional members alike engage in a discussion about the validity of the trial, attempting to distinguish between scientific merit and marketing claims. Nevertheless, CBTO's approach to informed consent by volunteers for HIV trials seems static. It assumes that once the informed-consent form is signed the volunteer has fully grasped its content. Certainly the IRB's approach to informed consent reflects a standard practice among boards at home and abroad.

> You know, there is an updated informed-consent form if things should change but from a legal standpoint the problem with the notion of the informed consent as not just an instance but as process is that if you say after you are in a trial "I understand it better now" then there is some suggestion that you understood it less before and then if you were understanding less, were you understanding so much less than you shouldn't have signed it to begin with. If so, all of the trial was unauthorized and that leaves you to the presence of liability. You have a mark in time, I see the liability from this moment forward. If you come back later and say, "OK, now I really understood" the first time was then unauthorized? And then it brings a lot of liability questions that make it crazy.
>
> I think that the informed-consent form is totally a legal document. The point of the informed consent is to be clear that there is a moment where you were given the option, yes, no, and you stated which your wishes are. (IRB's chair, 17 August 2004)

CBTO's IRB chair thus proposes that the legal character of the informed-consent form does not have a negative impact on volunteers' participation in the trials. On the contrary, she sees its legal character as protecting human subjects' rights, since violations of the informed-consent process can lead to stiff penalties and lawsuits against violators. "If in my desire, me meaning my pharmaceutical hat, if my desire to protect myself has the incidental benefit of making sure that you understand it, because if the only way that I get to be protected is if I explained it clearly to you, then good, everybody is happy" (IRB's chair, 17 August 2004). In addition, the IRB chair believes that the absence of conflicts of interest among its members ensures the independence of the board from industry pressures:

> We are a completely un-conflicted IRB. We are not benefiting from the research dollars given to CBTO. One member works for the AIDS library, which is a member of CBTO, but her salary and her position is not dependent upon CBTO getting research. As for the rest of us, we are separately employed, individual members of the community and thus we are not influenced by pharmaceutical dollars. In fact, my law firm does not accept pharmaceutical money. We don't solicit it, we don't accept it and so we try to be as—I don't want to say pure because then you have an indication that if you accept it you are not pure—but unbiased as possible.
>
> I think that if you compare us to other institutions' IRBs, where all the members are employed by the agency and where there is a direct correlation between the money in their pockets and the research they approve, compare that with our IRB where none of the members has a financial motivation to be on that board. You know, if CBTO stops doing research tomorrow, while it will be unfortunate for the community, it wouldn't affect me or anybody else on the board at all. And I think that the greatest protection for the patient comes from having a board that is completely conflict-free. So in this sense, we have been always conflict-free, we have been always mindful of having consumer participation, making sure that consumers on the board have an equal opportunity to evaluate risks and benefits.

One important function of the IRBs is to make sure that the informed-consent form follows standard guidelines for the protection of human subjects. The form should describe in lay terms the design, goals, risks, and benefits of the trial. It should be clear to the prospective volunteer that he or she can decline to participate or leave the trial at any time. Furthermore, alternative treatment options should be provided in case a volunteer decides not to join a trial.

The local IRB at CBTO goes to great lengths to ensure that these requirements are met in every informed-consent form submitted as part of the application for a new trial. However, the IRB is not supposed to, and does not, directly oversee the signing of the informed-consent form by patients, which is the responsibility of the principal investigator. At CBTO the principal investigator or head nurse is usually in charge to make sure that the procedures are followed.

The head nurse in charge of the SMART trial, one of the largest trials at CBTO, explains how she obtains informed consent from her patients: "As far as my patients go, every visit I go over the informed-consent form before the study begins reminding them what the study is about, reminding them what arm they were randomized to. I ask them if they have any questions. I tell them all the time that this is voluntary and I think that the patients in the SMART trial, anyway, they have a good understanding of it, as far as I know" (head nurse, 25 August 2004).

Although the informed-consent form follows certain legal standards, some trials have a more complex design than others, and this is reflected in the form. The SMART trial, for instance, randomized its population into two groups of volunteers; those in the first received their usual HIV medication while those in the second did not receive any medication unless their HIV defenses dropped below certain pre-established levels. The head nurse took great care in making sure that the patients enrolled in the trial understood abstract concepts like randomization, a key in the design of the trial. "They might not understand that word, that's why I use 'the flip of a coin.' They flip a coin and you can either get heads or tails and they I tell them what they mean. One is green, one is red, green means you go and red means that you stop, I try to make it in a language that they can understand. Plus we have a SMART media outlet that is very patient-friendly and has a good description of the informed-consent process, what the study is about, how long. They interview actual patients that have questions and then you can see on the tape, really nice" (head nurse, 25 August 2004).

As a result of these efforts CBTO staff seems confident that for the most part patients are aware of the trial's design, goals, risks, and benefits. Their PI summarizes this perspective: "The majority of patients that we had in trials understood what they were getting into. Some patients might have a slightly little understanding of what you would wish them to have, and usually you try to clarify that before they enter the trial, but I never encountered a patient that had an opposite understanding, or different understanding to the point they say: 'You know what, that is not what I thought it is.' I personally never had that experience, but it happens. I've heard that it happens."

ETHICS AND EXPLOITATION

Financial compensation for trial subjects has become an increasing presence in biomedicine, and clinical trials offer an additional venue for commodification of the body. Since the use of prisoners in trials research was banned in 1980, an expanding pharmaceutical industry has relied on market-recruited paid subjects to fill its needs. This shift has led to the emergence of a new class of professional guinea pig subjects. I will argue that the professionalization of trial subjects exploits a group of poor research subjects, subverting basic ethical principles and guidelines regulating the participation of human subjects in research.

On 12 July 1974 the National Research Act created the National Commission for the Protection of Human Subjects of Biomedical and Behavioral Research, and on 18 April 1979 the commission issued the Belmont Report. The report begins with a brief introduction to the ethical principles and guidelines for research involving human subjects, followed by a section setting the boundaries between practice and research. The following section outlines the main ethical principles: respect for the persons, beneficence, and justice. The final section outlines the application of these principles to the informed-consent process, the assessment of risk and benefit, and the selection of subjects.

The existence of market-recruited subjects in phase I clinical trials defies the principle of justice. According to the document an injustice occurs when "some benefit to which a person is entitled is denied without good reason or when some burden is imposed unduly" (1979, 5). Of course there is no mention to the professionalization of trial subjects, because it was not yet evident when the report was issued, but I would argue that the involvement of professional subjects in trial research is unjust because it burdens a group of poor research subjects without offering them a therapeutic benefit. Placing the burden of safety testing on professional guinea pigs seems also to contravene article 19 of the Declaration of Helsinki, which states that medical research is ethically justified only if there is a reasonable chance that the population in which it is conducted will benefit from the results.

Paid subjects fail to benefit from the research because they are healthy and have no need for the drugs they are testing, and also because, being unemployed or only partially employed, they are uninsured and would be unable to afford the drugs once they became available. The burden to research subjects is compounded by the inability of IRBs to monitor the participation of paid volunteers in phase I trials. IRBs are seldom able to make on-site inspections to verify trial conditions. This problem is more serious with IRBs "hired" by contract research organizations (CROs) to oversee pharmaceutical industry trials. As for the FDA, it usually inspects less than 1 percent of all clinical trials conducted in the country (Elliott and Abadie 2008). In addition, subjects who suffer injuries are not compensated for their pain and suffering or lost wages, although in some cases, like those of Ellen Roche and Jesse Gelsinger (an eighteen-year-old patient who died in 1998 after volunteering for a gene therapy trial at the University of Pennsylvania), legal settlements, usually out of court, have provided compensation to the families. For the most part, subjects cannot afford the legal assistance needed to fight for their rights, letting the pharmaceutical industry abuses go unchallenged.

Market recruitment has created a group of vulnerable research subjects, dependably and easily exploited. As this ethnography illustrates, trials are perceived as a business by the pharmaceutical industry and subjects alike. But the poverty of trial subjects and their dependence on trial income makes for their very unequal status vis-à-vis the pharmaceutical industry.

Money motivates subjects to enter the trials but is also used strategically by the industry to induce compliance. Participants are not paid in full unless they finish the trial—they may even receive a substantial bonus for completion—forcing subjects to accept harsh trial conditions, including risks higher than those they had expected. For participants who are not local residents and thus have incurred travel and housing expenses even before they were recruited, dropping out becomes harder than for local volunteers. By contrast, subjects living in areas with an abundant supply of trials can drop out of a trial—receiving a prorated compensation—and just as easily enroll in a more advantageous one. Anarchist guinea pigs living in West Philadelphia constitute in a way a privileged group of professional subjects. Very well informed and with a strong stand against the pharmaceutical industry, they are equipped with a healthy dose of cynicism and caution. But more importantly, with cheap rents available, no families to support, and low expenses, they can afford to wait for the best trial opportunities. That all of the anarchist guinea pigs whom I interviewed admitted volunteering at least once in a trial they thought was too risky or where working conditions were bad because they could not afford to drop out should give us reason for concern about the potential for further exploitation among other professional guinea pigs. For those who live in areas with fewer trial opportunities or who travel from one trial site to another in search of opportunities, incentives to enroll in a risky trial, to accept poor working conditions, or to remain in a trial despite possible secondary effects are much higher, placing them in a much more vulnerable position. And although rarer, the press has reported cases in which CROs have enrolled homeless and mentally ill persons, or illegal immigrants, into trials, offering the worst conditions imaginable.

While financial compensation does not necessarily make volunteers less well informed about a trial's goals, risks, and benefits, dependency on trial income interferes with the subjects' ability to freely consent to participate in research. The regulatory framework intended to protect human subjects, with ubiquitous IRBs and an emphasis on informed consent, was inspired by humanist values and in a reaction to Nazi abuses during the Second World War. However, my research illustrates that while the consent form is a necessary safeguard, IRB oversight of the informed-consent process may not be sufficient: it assumes a "free, uncoerced" subject that does not exist, and it focuses on informing subjects of the goals, risks, and benefits of a trial and not on policing the way the trial is carried out.

Despite these shortcomings, recent lawsuits have benefited patients and their families by taking aim at omissions and inaccuracies in the informed-consent process. As a result, companies and institutions are now better aware of the wording of their consent forms, which include carefully crafted disclaimers. Of course, this language only obscures the risks and benefits of clinical trials to participants.

LIVING IN/OFF THE MILD TORTURE
ECONOMY AS TRIAL SUBJECTS

By following the commodity chain from "first-in-man" phase I trials to phase III, I explored the relationship between the increasing commodification of volunteers' participation in clinical trials and its effects on the way risk is constructed and managed. My work illustrates how the market recruitment of trial subjects has led to a process of professionalization among volunteers, signaled by the emergence of a group of professional guinea pigs who provide the pharmaceutical industry with a regular supply of healthy, disciplined bodies it needs to run an increasing number of phase I trials. The prospect of "easy, quick money" is enough to motivate mainly poor, unemployed working-class people to enter into the "economy of the flesh" by becoming trial subjects. This constitutes just another turn in the increasing commodification of the body in biomedical research, along with the maintenance of a market for body organs and parts. While volunteers are deeply aware of the commodification of their bodies, this fact is denied by the pharmaceutical industry.

The pharmaceutical industry denies commodification by employing a series of semantic turns to portray subjects as "paid volunteers" being compensated for their time and effort. However, paid subjects become aware of their status not as volunteers but as workers, and develop a shared identity based on common experiences and interests. Professional guinea pigs find ways to express their opposition to the commodification of their bodies and the conditions that dehumanize, alienate, and exploit them. Everyday forms of resistance include refusal to follow diet regimes and attempts to disrupt trial results. The volunteers' successful strike at

Jefferson shows not only the potential for collective action but also the limits imposed by their mobility and fragmentation.

The commodification of the subjects' bodies entails continuous participation in trial research, exposing professional guinea pigs to risks they might be unable or unwilling to recognize. Market recruitment shapes the subjects' understanding of risk and also their responses to it. Their perception as "contractors" being hired for individual trials made professional subjects consider the risks in the trials they were joining, but they did not consider the cumulative result of drug interactions resulting from years of trial participation. Furthermore, the compensation on which the subjects depended to sustain their lifestyles seemed to predispose them to neglect the effects of long-term participation in clinical trials. To complicate their situation, when evaluating risk, volunteers constructed a scale that placed certain trials, like those involving psychiatric drugs and other drugs perceived to be especially dangerous, at the top of the scale, but in practice financial inducements still lead them to volunteer for trials that they consider high-risk. All subjects admitted having done at least one trial that they considered too risky because the money was too good to refuse. Some might attempt to drop out of a particular trial if adverse effects seemed more serious than expected, but doing so entails a financial loss and therefore is not a common practice.

Unlike coal miners, asbestos workers, and other employees working in toxic environments, trial volunteers are mobile and work sporadically, making it more difficult for them to share information about side effects, especially over the long term. Also, neither the pharmaceutical industry nor the FDA keeps careful records of the frequency and type of clinical trials, making the monitoring of effects still more difficult.

While financial compensation is also offered to patients at CBTO who volunteer to test HIV drugs, this reward cannot be compared to the sums received in phase I research. For HIV trial volunteers money is not the main inducement, nor does it shape their identities or their experiences of the trial. The narratives of John, Geraldine, and Michael show that the decision to volunteer for HIV trials is part of their struggle against the disease. The trial offered them the opportunity to gain valuable knowledge about the workings of the virus, their health status, and for Michael, an opportunity to expand therapies after years of dealing with the disease.

Chapter 7 shows that commodification shapes the way professional guinea pigs perceive and respond to the informed-consent form. For this group the form provoked anxieties about the exploitation and dehumanization that they experienced as paid human subjects. In particular, the anarchist professional guinea pigs demonstrated a research ethic that differed from that of the scientific community. As a result of their hostility toward the pharmaceutical industry, they felt the need to become active agents in evaluating the information in the informed-consent form. Based on their own history as research subjects they also felt that they had something to contribute to the role of human subjects in drug research.

For HIV patients at CBTO the informed-consent form elicited a response characterized not by distrust to the scientific establishment but by their confidence and trust in doctors. Finally, for their local IRB and for the scientific staff, the possibility of conducting "industry" trials (in contrast to "community trials") represented both an opportunity and a danger. Industry trials might contribute to the development of much-needed new drug therapies that could improve the quality of life for patients. On the other hand, CBTO is a community-based organization, and pressure from financial interests was a concern. A "totally un-conflicted IRB" was perceived to be a safeguard against undue pressures from industry. In addition, lay and professional members engaged in formal discussions in relation to the informed-consent process, concerning the validity of the trial design. They were suspicious of any trial that was only intended to advance "marketing claims." However, the tensions between the demands of the industry trials and CBTO's commitment to HIV patients only increase along with the number of pharmaceutical trials.

The commodification of clinical-trials research and in particular of phase I studies exposes volunteers to new and unexpected risks resulting from continuous participation and also challenges major ethical principles and guidelines to protect human subjects in research. The shift from a captive population to a market-recruited population unfairly targets a particular socioeconomic group, creating a new type of captive and vulnerable population. This contradiction with ethical norms and regulations is masked by existing notions of an autonomous, free individual able to "contract" in a way that previous groups of captive populations were not. This legalistic view of the encounter between the paid subject and the industry is incorporated into the informed-consent form, which has become a legal document that confuses and alienates research subjects.

The emergence of professional guinea pigs in phase I trials research in the United States parallels the emergence of a globalized and flexible model of capital accumulation over the last two decades. Political theorists like Nikolas Rose and Graham Burchell (1991) show how these new regimes of capital accumulation have emerged in conjunction with new neoliberal rationalities of rule that transform citizens' subjectivities. Rose illustrates the "enhancement of the powers of the client as customer-consumer of health services, of education, of training etc. which specifies the subjects of rule in a new way: as active subjects individuals seeking to 'enterprise themselves,' to maximize their quality of life through choice, according their life a meaning and value to the extent that it can be rationalized as the outcomes of the choices made" (1996, 57). According to Rose, "this notion of the neo-liberal governance requiring that the goals of the state and individuals being the same, assumes that people make a role in "enterprising" themselves, in the name of personal freedom and freedom of choice" (Rose 1996). This new, entrepreneurial self becomes thus functional to the interests of the neoliberal state, which can now rely on economizing to serve the interests of global capital.

Professional guinea pigs embody the new subjectivity required by neoliberal governmentality. Their flexible bodies (Martin 1994), disciplined, compliant, yet with open schedules and high geographical mobility come handy and "ready-made" to serve the needs of a regional and global economy. Their desire for this kind of work and lifestyle makes of these subjects the most flexible workers imaginable, constituting the prototypical "footsoldiers of global capital" (Mitchell 2003).

This might be the ultimate irony for the anarchist research subjects. Their entrepreneurism as "self-contractors" constitutes not a withdrawal from a system they despise but a fundamental goal of neoliberal governmentality. While they think they are "opting out" of the system by becoming guinea pigs, they do not realize that their ability to do so depends on a neoliberal economy.

It is a neoliberal imperative for individuals to feel that they are making their own choices and for them to take responsibility for their own actions, in particular actions that may place them at risk. As my research has shown, informed-consent forms make research subjects responsible for their own decisions while obscuring possible risks by semantic turns and technical language. I believe in the need to move beyond neoliberal frameworks that emphasize individual responsibility for risks and replace them with a deeper understanding of how corporate desires, technological advances, and neoliberal regimes of governance place certain groups at risk as research subjects.

The continuous development of a population of professional research subjects demands an anthropological exploration of the ethical ramifications of the increasing commodification of the body in clinical-trials research. I am aware that my work may challenge powerful interests that will try to discredit my main arguments and findings. Some may dismiss the role of professional guinea pigs in the current organization of phase I trials as a very small, unrepresentative minority, in contrast to the many volunteers who have only altruistic motives. Yet as this book illustrates, far from being a rare, exotic specimen, professional guinea pigs form the backbone of the healthy, paid population that tests drug safety in America. Without their disciplined, compliant bodies, no trial would be possible. Despite the industry's denials, healthy, paid subjects have become valuable commodities, since the pharmaceutical companies are now dependent on poor, vulnerable, easily exploited subjects to fill their phase I trials. Market-recruitment proved to be—at least from the perspective of the pharmaceutical industry—a successful way of filling their need for trial subjects. How else could the industry find a population willing to volunteer in their trials? After all, not everyone wishes to test the toxicity of drugs that he or she does not need, while subjected to uncomfortable procedures and degrading working conditions.

This book demonstrates that guinea-pigging is not a fashion, esoteric culture, or favored lifestyle. Professional guinea pigs are not an oddity or, as someone suggested to me, a pathology, of clinical trials research, but the product of pharmaceutical industry requirements. Pharmaceutical research feeds on a mass of destitute citizens who realized that clinical trials offered a better opportunity than jobs at McDonald's and similar dead-end options at the bottom of the new, service-oriented economy.

Of course, as I have mentioned, the anarchist guinea pigs living in West Philly are only a very small part of the universe of professional research subjects. While their views on the politics and ethics of trials research and their perspectives on the roles of the pharmaceutical industry and the state might not be shared by other professional guinea pigs, they all have the same motivations and experiences as trial subjects, which their metaphorical identification with guinea pigs illustrates. They are all subjected to the same routines, pain, boredom, and risks. All reaffirm their human condition and decry the dehumanizing, impersonal treatment they receive as trial subjects.

I am not suggesting an absence of differences between professional guinea pigs in America. Even the small group of anarchist guinea pigs is far from homogeneous. Anarchist women whom I interviewed seemed to be a little ashamed of their trial participation and critical of their male anarchist counterparts for placing their health in danger while also helping the pharmaceutical industry profit though drug development.

Recently I read a piece in the *New York Times* about a group of college students at a Catholic university in the Midwest who had resorted to clinical trials to earn enough money to pay their increasing tuition costs. That alone would not be unusual: students continue to provide a steady supply of trial subjects. What surprised me was that these volunteers from a very Catholic college had struggled with the notion that guinea-pigging was "unnatural" and therefore would be a sin before deciding that God would forgive them for their guinea-pigging. Stories like this one provide hints into the multiple realities behind the professionalization of trials subjects.

We are only beginning to approach an anthropological understanding of paid research subjects in phase I trials. This ethnography is the first step in that direction. The white male anarchists from West Philadelphia who are the subject of this book constitute a very visible and relevant section of the professional guinea pig population, but they are numerically a tiny minority. Most trials in the city run without any of them: at any given moment not more than two or three of them will be involved in any trial. And they rarely venture to do trials outside the Philadelphia metropolitan area. While providing an invaluable window into professionalization among phase I subjects, they also took pains to remind me that professional guinea pigs are a very heterogeneous group, although united by similar experiences and interests as trial subjects.

We need to extend the study into other groups: college students in need of tuition money, the underemployed and unemployed, even unemployable ex-prisoners allegedly being enrolled right out of jail in New

Jersey, or undocumented Latinos making a living as trial subjects in Florida (Elliott and Abadie 2008). As the current economic crisis worsens, more groups will be tempted to become trial subjects, raising new questions of race, class, ethics, compliance, exploitation, and agency.

African Americans have been historically wary of biomedical research —for good reason—and their apprehension continues today, with lower recruitment rates even for diseases that disproportionately affect them, like HIV and diabetes. Still, poor African Americans constitute an important resource in phase I trials and are regularly recruited by the industry. How do they overcome their misgivings and suspicions to enroll in the trials? What is their experience in the trials and how do they talk about it? Is there something unique about their trial participation when compared with other groups of professional guinea pigs? And finally, what does the participation of the poor, from African American and other ethnic backgrounds, say not about them but about ourselves, the kind of society we live in and the choices we make to assess the safety of the drugs we consume?

No ethnographic inquiry of phase I clinical trials should let the pharmaceutical industry off the hook. I had initially contacted a senior researcher at a very large pharmaceutical firm regarding the way management thought about risks and financial compensation in clinical trials. The researcher was a trained epidemiologist and had worked for the city of Philadelphia for many years before taking up his current position, in which he is in charge of post-marketing surveillance. If any adverse effects showed after a drug was on the market, he had to assess whether they were related to the drug, whether they were serious if they were related, and how management should deal with the problem.

We met in a park once and had a nice conversation. I remember his telling me that if a company suspected any safety concerns associated with a drug during clinical trials it would immediately address them, because it was the right thing to do but also because the company stood to lose millions if the same problem showed up years later when the drug was on the market and had to be withdrawn. Unfortunately the researcher was very busy and we never managed to meet again. I wanted to ask him about the withdrawal of the painkiller Vioxx from the market in 2004 after it was demonstrated that the drug was not more effective than those already in the market and presented an unacceptable risk of heart attacks. Lawsuits showed that Merck knew of these problems all along and did its best to neglect them. I am still hopeful. However, the traditional secrecy surrounding the pharmaceutical industry can be breached in other, more indirect ways. The Vioxx trial offers valuable opportunities to explore issues of risk, profit, drug approval regulations, and consumers' health. Lawsuits are opening a trove of industry documents, memos, e-mail messages, and trial protocols. In addition, some scientists and regulators at the Food and Drug Administration are offering their views on these issues. And the pharmaceutical industry is not only one of the biggest industries but also one of the most globalized. Its global character opens opportunities for comparative studies of pharmaceutical practices and governmental regulation in clinical-trials research.

CAN PUBLIC POLICY PROTECT PROFESSIONAL RESEARCH SUBJECTS?

One of the strengths of ethnographic research is its ability to provide a rich, textured description of a phenomenon. At its best, it enables informants' voices, analyzed and placed in the proper context, to provide insight into groups' views and experiences while affirming our shared humanity and questioning deeply held societal assumptions about who we are and how we live. But I also hope that by describing the articulation of scientific, medical, social, and economic practices that make possible the participation of human subjects in trials research, this book will stimulate debate and bring about public policies that are better able to protect research subjects.

Risk is an inherent part of biomedical research and of phase I trials in particular. While some compounds tested in phase I trials have already been approved and tested by millions of consumers, others are experimental and have only been tried in dogs and rats. That subjects receive doses much larger than those consumed by the public once the drug is approved only compounds the risk they face.

Can public policy protect professional research subjects? Eliminating phase I trials is not an option, because doing so would only transfer the risk to later phases in trials research and to the overall population who would later consume the drugs. Maintaining phase I trials but ending financial compensation so that all volunteers were altruistic would not work either. This solution might be appealing but would considerably slow down or stop drug development altogether. After all, asking citizens to place themselves in harm's way by taking drugs they do not need to assess their toxicity might be quite a duty call for most. Not to mention that even very altruistic subjects might be hesitant to volunteer to test drugs for a pharmaceutical industry that they might perceive as not trustworthy. Altruism would also deprive poor research subjects of much-needed income.

Since reliance on paid professional trial subjects seems to be the best alternative, at least for the time being, the following recommendations aim not to eliminate risk—they could not have avoided the deaths of Ellen Roche, Jesse Gelsinger, and others—but to minimize it while also making risk more transparent and explicit. A related goal is to address the exploitation and abuse of trial subjects by making sure that their rights as subjects, as well as the rights of workers, are respected. Of course some recommendations, in particular regarding limits on the number of trials conducted, or on the number of trials that a volunteer can join, directly challenge current pharmaceutical arrangements and interests and will be very hard to implement.

The first recommendation is to keep detailed records documenting the participation of paid volunteers in trials research. Of particular relevance is information about the identity of volunteers, as well as how often, where, and in which trials they participate. Data about ADRs and other events should also be recorded. The best way of implementing this recommendation would be to create a centralized register. The FDA would be a good place to house a register if it decides to overcome its current timidity about overseeing the conditions in which paid subjects volunteer for phase I trials. This recommendation would also enhance the accountability of the pharmaceutical industry and its CROs and should be paired with the elimination of industry-hired IRBs, which should be replaced by publicly funded review boards.

This point relates to the next recommendation: the need to carry out scientific, impartial studies of possible drug interactions over the short term and long term, to document and prevent long-term toxicity and synergistic effects.

We also need to recognize that volunteers' participation is labor, even if it is what they call a "weird type of work," and provide better working conditions and proper compensation. Paid subjects should be given the same labor protections guaranteed to other workers in risky occupations.

Subjects may have a role to play in regulating working conditions as well. They could create a publicly accessible register of trial sites where subjects are able to evaluate conditions in different facilities, from the quality of the staff to the food to other items of interest to participants. Report cards similar to those published in *Guinea Pig Zero* would be a good start. However, implementing this recommendation would engage volunteers in a much larger and more sustained effort than they might be willing to undertake.

The last recommendation—and the most difficult to implement—is to restrict the number of trials, thus diminishing drug exposure and potential adverse effects. Since this would alter the market-based organization of trials research, it could encounter stiff resistance from the pharmaceutical industry. However, from the point of view of larger social interests there is no harm involved in this measure. Most trials are conducted on "me-too drugs"—versions of drugs that are already in the market. This increases the industry's profits, allowing them to extend patent protection and capture or expand market share, while exposing volunteers to risk with no scientific advancement. One way to achieve this recommendation would be by taxing "me-too" trials while providing tax incentives for trials that test new, experimental drugs.

There are obstacles. Currently the Food and Drug Administration is more interested in facilitating a good business climate than in public intervention, and it might not want to implement these recommendations. In addition, some recommendations challenge the industry's dependence upon paid research subjects in phase I clinical drug trials. Finally, the subjects themselves might not endorse policy recommendations that might limit their ability to enroll in trials, even if it benefited them in the long run.

FOLLOWING UP

Robert Helms, Frank Little, Dave Onion, and Spam One Last Time

One of the advantages—or disadvantages—of doing fieldwork at home is that one never effectively leaves. Once I finished my fieldwork in Philadelphia I moved back to New York City. I wrote my dissertation and left for the Midwest for an academic appointment. But in all these years I kept in contact, basically through e-mail, with guinea pigs in West Philadelphia. In March 2008 I decided to go back once more for a final round of interviews. I wanted to know what they had been doing since the last time I had seen them, get some sense of the guinea pig scene in the city, and inquire about their future plans and aspirations. The meetings were very informal, more a friendly reunion than a research occasion; I didn't dare take out my tape recorder. My fieldwork notes provide a sense of our conversations. This final wandering into the trajectories of a group of professional guinea pigs provides another glimpse into their lives in the context of an ever-changing neighborhood, city, and trial economy.

I met Robert Helms at 10:00 am at his place, 45th and Baltimore. It was a neat house with a wooden porch. He lived with a roommate and five cats (two were his). He was very proud of his black cat, recently portrayed along with Helms in the magazine *Wired*. He showed me the picture along with the article about the anarchist guinea pigs in Philadelphia. We walked up Baltimore Avenue to a café on 49th street, just across Fancy House, where I had lived during fieldwork. I could immediately see how much the area had changed since I left. Pointing to the locale of the Industrial Workers of the World (IWW), now with a bookstore in the front, Helms explained that they were still functioning but had moved to a back room. The space also hosted poetry events. Café Africa had closed, replaced by an upscale café. The café we were heading to on 49th street was just below the Firehouse bike shop and was also new. It was crowded, organic, alternative, and mostly white. The food market on the corner was also gone: a trendy bar had taken over, but since it was early in the morning it had not opened yet. We went back to a pizza place on 45th and got some beers. Helms told me that after I saw him in Paris he finished doing research for a movie about the cult murders in Georgetown, Guyana, for a Canadian company—the movie went on the market with the title *Paradise Lost*—then hung around for a little bit and came back to Philadelphia in June 2005. He stayed abroad for twenty months.

Once back in the city he sustained himself by painting houses, as he had done before. He told me he had quite a bit of work now, with all these new people moving in and buying property in the area. He had stopped doing trials when he made forty-five, which is the age limit for most trials, and now was not very "active." He had updated the *Guinea Pig Zero* site a few times, most recently six or eight months ago, and had enjoyed quite a bit of attention lately since Carl Elliott's article in the *New Yorker* directly mentioned him. Just last week someone from Stanford University visited him, and Dan Rather's producer had contacted him as well. I asked him if he missed doing trials. He told me not really, the money was good but trials were incredibly boring.

Helms had three book deals. He would not make any money, he told me, because he chose small, independent presses or web publication. All three books were historical and biographical explorations about nineteenth-century anarchists. Just a couple of days earlier he had started working as a labor organizer in health care, which was his old profession. He was very enthusiastic about this new job. He would be paid to organize health care workers but could work in health care as well on the side, doubling his salary.

I wanted to have a sense of the guinea pig crowd in Philadelphia and of the trials in the city. I was under the impression that after GSK closed its facility other companies had followed, leaving few opportunities for guinea-pigging. Helms told me I was wrong. Yes, GSK closed, but another business took over (he thinks it was a CRO). Wyeth was still doing trials, and he thought that Merck was too, at Jefferson. There was a new site as well. He suggested that I talk with Frank Little, who was still active. I told him I was planning to do so.

Helms mentioned that Spam had moved just a few blocks away, to a house he had bought, and was still working as a janitor organizer, although for a different union. He had seen him last Thursday at an event organized to discuss working conditions in the maquiladoras in Mexico. He saw Dave Onion there. He was still living in his house but was not doing trials any more. Helms was not sure what Dave Onion was doing for a living but told me that he now wore a very large, red beard, like a nineteenth-century anarchist.

I joined Frank Little at Café Vientiane, just between the Mariposa Co-op and Dalhak bar. These shops had not been altered that much; still, talk about how much the neighborhood had changed was unavoidable. Frank told me that it had gentrified quite a bit, and apparently anarchists in the area had targeted the new bar on the corner of 49th street as a symbol of the process. He found this opposition misguided—the beer was quite good, he assured me—and also, the Catholic church across the street had also opposed the bar, giving him pause. He was uneasy with the idea that the church and the anarchist community would come together to protest.

The last time Frank and I had met was right before the presidential elections. Since elections were now coming, he told me that it must have been four years since our last meeting. In the meantime he had traveled to Cambodia, Vietnam, and Thailand for four months with the money he had received from two inpatient trials (around five to six thousand dollars). That was two years ago or so. He was not doing inpatient trials that much now. Frank still derived two-thirds of his income from trials but preferred to do outpatient trials, usually at the University of Pennsylvania, things like computer tests that paid $75, or he would sell white blood cells for $150. Once a year he considered doing an inpatient trial if his schedule permitted. He told me he could live on $20 a day (the cost of monthly rent and utilities in his communal housing was $300) and that it was not hard to get by. He supplemented his income by doing odd jobs that he found through Craigslist. Most of his time was spent on political activism. When I first met him the antiwar rallies kept him very busy. Now he dedicated his time to other political causes and helped Dave Onion edit the *Defenestrator*, which is still being published.

Coming back to a topic he had explored with me in earlier conversations, Frank told me that he didn't envision himself being a volunteer all his life. He had already significantly reduced the number of trials he volunteered for. He told me that life in West Philadelphia was nice and easy—doing political activism, hanging around, travels funded by trials money—but he did not want to do it forever, although sometimes he feared that he might have to if he let his guard down. Frank told me he would like to explore being a merchant marine or go back to school and become a schoolteacher, probably in New York City.

As for other trial subjects beyond the anarchist community, which he emphatically pointed out to me accounted for the large majority of participants—sometimes he was the only white participant in a trial—he said that sometimes he asked them if they intended to do trials forever but that "they don't want to think about it." This answer immediately reminded me of the way anarchist guinea pigs answered my own questions about the possibility of adverse drug reactions and long-term effects.

Frank has also been courted by journalists. They were up for sensationalistic coverage, he told me, and ignored his claims that nothing exceptional happened in trials: they are a business, they are boring, and white anarchists are a drop in the bucket. He encouraged me to do more research and volunteered to put me in touch with African American guinea pigs conducting trials in the city. Frank even volunteered to hook me up in a trial site. We agreed that I should join one as part of my next research project. Finally, I asked him about changes in the trial scene. He said that GSK had closed but was bought by Astrazeneca, which occupied the same spot inside the Penn campus, close to Presbyterian Hospital. He mentioned that the firm had brought in a new, large plasma TV and pool tables and kept some of the former personnel. Anarchists that move into the area and other professional guinea pigs have no trouble getting into trials. This mild torture economy seems to be as strong as ever.

BIBLIOGRAPHY

Abadie, Roberto. 2008. "The Ethics Debate on Compensating Drug Trial Volunteers." *Anthropology News*, February, 24.

———. 2009. "A Guinea Pig's Wage: Risk and Commoditization in Clinical Trials Drug Research in America." *Killer Commodities: A Critical Anthropological Examination of Corporate Products and Public Health*, ed. Merrill Singer and Hans Baer. New York: Rowman and Littlefield.

Abraham, John. 1994. *Science, Politics and the Pharmaceutical Industry*. London: UCL Press.

Abraham, John, and John Sheppard. 1997. "Democracy, Technocracy and the Secret State of Medicines Control: Expert and Non-expert Perspectives." *Science, Technology, and Human Values* 22, 139–67.

Adams, Carolyn, ed. 1991. *Philadelphia: Neighborhoods, Division, and Conflict in a Postindustrial City*. Philadelphia: Temple University Press.

Ajzen, I., and M. Fishbein, eds. 1980. *Understanding Attitudes and Predicting Social Behaviors*. Englewood Cliffs, N.J.: Prentice-Hall.

Altman, Lawrence K. 2001. "U.S. to Investigate Death in an Asthma Study." *New York Times*, 16 June, A, 13.

Altman, Robert. 1998. *Who Goes First? The Story of Self-experimentation in Medicine*. Berkeley: University of California Press.

Andrews, Dorothy, and Dorothy Nelkin. 2004. *Body Bazaar: The Market for Human Tissue in the Biotechnology Age*. New York: Crown.

Angell, Marcia. 2004. *The Truth about the Drug Companies: How They Deceive Us and What to Do about It*. New York: Random House.

Annas, George, and Michael H. Grodin. 1992. *The Nazi Doctors and the Nuremberg Code: Human Rights in Experimentation*. New York: Oxford University Press.

Appadurai, Arjun, ed. 1986. *The Social Life of Things: Commodities in Cultural Perspective*. Cambridge: Cambridge University Press.

Arendt, Hannah. 1958. *The Human Condition*. Chicago: University of Chicago Press.

Arno, Peter S., and Karyn L. Feiden. 1992. *Against the Odds: The Story of AIDS Drug Development, Politics and Profits*. New York: Harper Collins.

Asad, Talal. 1996. "On Torture, or Cruel, Inhuman, and Degrading Treatment." *Social Suffering*, ed. A. Kleinman, V. Das, and M. Lock, 285–308. Berkeley: University of California Press.

Associated Press. 2006. "6 Fall Seriously Ill during Drug Test in London." 16 March.

Baer, Hans. 1992. Review of *The Politics of Public Health*. *Medical Anthropology Quarterly*, n.s. 6, no. 2, 176–78.

———. 2001. *Biomedicine and Alternative Healing Systems in America: Issues of Class, Race, Ethnicity, and Gender*. Madison: University of Wisconsin Press.

Baer, Hans, Merrill Singer, and Ida Susser. 2003. *Medical Anthropology and the World System*. 2nd edn. Westport, Conn.: Praeger.

Balis, Andrea. 2000. "Miracle Medicine: The Impact of Sulfa Drugs on Medicine, in Pharmaceutical Industry and Govermental Regulations in the U.S. in the 1930s." Diss., Graduate Center, City University of New York.

Barber, Bernard. 1973. *Research on Human Subjects: Problems of Social Control in Medical Experimentation*. New York, Russell Sage Foundation.

———. 1980. *Informed Consent in Medical Therapy and Research*. New Brunswick, N.J.: Rutgers University Press.

Beardsley, Edward. 1987. *A History of Neglect: Health Care for Blacks and Mill Workers in the Twentieth-Century South*. Knoxville: University of Tennessee Press.

Beck, Ullrich. 1992. *Risk Society: Towards a New Modernity*. London: Sage.

Beck, Ullrich, Anthony Giddens, and Scott Lash. 1994. *Reflexive Modernization: Politics, Tradition and Aestheticism in the Modern Social Order*. Cambridge: Polity.

Becker, H. S., et al. 1976. *Boys in White: Student Culture in Medical School*. Chicago: University of Chicago Press.

Becker, Marshall, and Jill Joseph. 1988. "Aids and Behavioral Changes to Avoid Risk: A Review." *American Journal of Public Health* 78, 384–410.

Beecher, Henry. 1966. "Ethics and Clinical Research." *New England Journal of Medicine* 274, no. 24 (June), 1354–60.

———. 1995. "Experimentation in Man." *Journal of the American Medical Association* 169, 461–78.

Bellaby, Paul. 1990. "To Risk or Not to Risk? Uses and Limitations of Mary Douglas on Risk-Acceptability for Understanding Health and Safety at Work and Road Accidents." *Sociological Review* 38, 465–83.

Bentar, Solomon. 2000. "Distributive Justice and Clinical Trials in the Third World." *Theoretical Medicine and Bioethics* 22, no. 3, 169–76.

Berman, Marshall. 1982. *All That Is Solid Melts into Air: The Experience of Modernity*. New York: Simon and Schuster.

Biehl, Joao. 2007. *Will to Live: AIDS Therapies and the Politics of Survival*. Princeton: Princeton University Press.

Biehl, Joao, Denise Coutinho, and Ana Luiza Outeiro. 2003. "Technology and Affect: HIV/AIDS Testing in Brazil." *Culture, Medicine and Psychiatry* 25, no. 1, 87–129.

Blim, Michael. 1992. *Studies of the New Industrialization in the Late Twentieth Century*. New York: Praeger.

———. 2005. *Equality and Economy: The Global Challenge.* Walnut Creek, Calif.: AltaMira.

Bloor, Michael. 1995. "Theories of HIV Related Risk Behavior." *Medicine, Health and Risk*, ed. J. Gabe. London: Blackwell.

Bluestone, D., and B. Harrison. 1982. *The Deindustrialization of America: Plant Closing, Community Abandonment, and the Dismantling of Basic Industry.* New York: Basic.

Bosk, Charles. 2000. "Irony, Ethnography, and Informed Consent." *Bioethics in Social Context*, ed. Barry Hoffmaster. Philadelphia: Temple University Press.

———. 2005. *What Would You Do? The Collision of Ethnography and Ethics.* Chicago: University of Chicago Press.

Bourgeois, Philippe. 2004. *In Search of Respect: Selling Crack in El Barrio.* Cambridge: Cambridge University Press.

Brandt, Allan. 1987. *No Magic Bullet: A Social History of Venereal Disease in the United States since 1880.* New York: Oxford University Press.

Burawoy, Michael. 1979. *Manufacturing Consent: Changes in the Labor Process under Monopoly Capitalism.* Chicago: University of Chicago Press.

Burchell, Graham, Gordon Colin, and Peter Miller, eds. 1991. *The Foucault Effect: Studies in Governmentality.* Chicago: University of Chicago Press.

Callahan, D. 1999. "The Social Sciences and the Task of Bioethics." *Daedalus* 128, no. 4, 275–94.

Clatts, M., S. Deren, and S. Friedman. 1989. "La construction sociale du Sida chez les consommateurs de drogue à Harlem." *Anthropologie et sociétés* 15, 37–59.

Connors, M. 1996. "Risk Perception, Risk Taking and Risk Management among Intravenous Drug Users: Implications for Drug Prevention." *Social Science and Medicine* 34, 591–601.

Corrigan, Oonagh P. 2002. "A Risky Business: The Detection of Adverse Drug Reactions in Clinical Trials and Post-Marketing Exercises." *Social Science and Medicine* 55, 497–507.

Csordas, Thomas. 1994. *Embodiment and Experience: The Existential Ground of Culture and Self.* New York: Cambridge University Press.

Darvall, Leanna. 1993. *Medicine, Law and Social Change: The Impact of Bioethics, Feminism and Rights Movements in Medical Decision-Making.* Aldershot: Darmouth.

Das, Veena. 1999. "Public Good, Ethics, and Everyday Life: Beyond the Boundaries of Bioethics." *Daedalus* 128 (fall), 99–134.

Davis, Mike. 1990. *City of Quartz: Excavating the Future of Los Angeles.* New York: Verso.

Dean, M. 1999. "Risk, Calculable or Incalculable." *Risk and Socio-cultural Theory: New Directions and Perspectives*, ed. D. Lupton. Cambridge: Cambridge University Press.

de Certau, Michael. 1982. *The Practice of Everyday Life.* Berkeley: University of California Press.

di Leonardo, Michaela. 1998. *Exotics at Home: Anthropologies, Others, American Modernity.* Chicago: University of Chicago Press.

Douglas, Mary. 1970. *Natural Symbols.* London: Cresset.

———. 1981. "De la souillure." *Essai sur les notions de pollution et taboo.* London: Maspero.

———. 1992. *Risk and Blame: Essays in Cultural Theory.* London: Routledge.

Douglas, M., and A. Wildavsky. 1981. *Risk and Culture*. Berkeley: University of California Press.

Edwards, Sarah, Richard Lilford, J. Thornton, and J. Hewison. 1997. "Informed Consent for Clinical Trials: In Search of the 'Best' Method." *Social Science Medicine* 47, no. 11, 1825–40.

Elliott, Carl. 2006. "The Drug Pushers." *Atlantic Monthly*, April, 2–13.

———. 2008. "Guinea-Pigging: Healthy Human Subjects for Drug-Safety Trials Are in Demand. But, Is It a Living?" *New Yorker*, January, 36–41.

Elliott, Carl, and Roberto Abadie. 2008. "Exploiting a Research Underclass in Phase I Clinical Trials." *New England Journal of Medicine* 358, no. 22, 2316–17.

Epstein, Steven. 1996. *Impure Science: AIDS, Activism, and the Politics of Knowledge*. Berkeley: University of California Press.

Etkin, N. L. 1992. "Side Effects: Cultural Constructions and Reinterpretations of Western Pharmaceuticals." *Medical Anthropology Quarterly* 6, 99–113.

Evans-Pritchard, Evans. 1980. *Witchcraft, Oracles, and Magic among the Azande*. Oxford: Clarendon.

Faden, Ruth, and Tom L. Beauchamp. 1986. *Theory of Informed Consent*. New York: Oxford University Press.

Farmer, Paul. 1992. *AIDS and Accusation: Haiti and the Geography of Blame*. Berkeley: University of California Press.

———. 2001. *Infections and Inequalities: The Modern Plagues*. Berkeley: University of California Press.

———. 2002. *Pathologies of Power: Health, Human Rights, and the New War on the Poor*. Berkeley: University of California Press.

Farmer, Paul, Margaret Connors, and Janie Simmons, eds. 1996. *Women, Poverty, and AIDS: Sex, Drugs, and Structural Violence*. Monroe, Maine: Common Courage.

Fisher, Jill. 2009. *Medical Research for Hire: The Political Economy of Pharmaceutical Clinical Trials*. New Brunswick, N.J.: Rutgers University Press.

Fisher, Michael. 2003. *Emergent Forms of Life and the Anthropological Voice*. Durham: Duke University Press.

Fox, Renee. 1961. "Physicians on the Drug Industry Side of the Prescription Blank: Their Dual Commitment to Medical Science and Business." *Journal of Health and Human Behavior* 2, no. 1 (spring), 3–16.

———. 1974. *Experiment Perilous: Physicians and Patients Facing the Unknown*. Philadelphia: University of Pennsylvania Press.

———. 1976. "Advanced Medical Technologies: Social and Ethical Implications." *Annual Review of Sociology* 2, 231–68.

———. 1997. "The Evolution of American Bioethics: A Sociological Perspective." *Social Science Perspectives on Medical Ethics*, ed. George Weisz, 201–20. Philadelphia: University of Pennsylvania Press.

Franklin, Sarah. 1995. "Science as Culture, Cultures of Science." *Annual Review of Anthropology*, 163–342.

Freund, Paul A. 1970. *Experimentation with Human Beings*. New York: George Braziller.

Garret, Leslie. 2000. *Betrayal of Trust: The Collapse of Global Public Health*. New York: Hyperion.

Giddens, Anthony. 1990. *The Consequences of Modernity*. Stanford: Sanford University Press.

Goffman, Erving. 1961. *Asylums: Essays on the Social Situation of Mental Patients and Other Inmates*. Garden City, N.Y: Anchor.

Goode, Judith, and Jo Anne Schneider. 1994. *Reshaping Ethnic Relations in Philadelphia: Immigrants in a Divided City*. Philadelphia: Temple University Press.

Gray, Bradford H. 1975. *Human Subjects in Medical Experimentation*. New York: John Wiley and Sons.

Gutman, Herbert. 1975. *Work, Culture and Society in Industrializing America: Essay in America Working Class and Social History*. New York: Alfred A. Knopf.

Hackings, Ian. 1990. *The Taming of Chance*. Cambridge: Cambridge University Press.

Harkness, Jon. 1996. "Nuremberg and the Issue of Wartime Experiments on U.S. Prisoners." *Journal of the American Medical Association* 276, no. 20, 1672–75.

Harrington, Anne. 1997. *The Placebo Effect: An Interdisciplinary Exploration*. Cambridge: Harvard University Press.

Hartman, Chester. 1997. *Double Exposure: Poverty and Race in America*. New York: M. E. Sharpe.

Harvey, David. 2002. *The New Imperialism*. Oxford: Oxford University Press, 2002.

Healy, David. 2004. *Let Them Eat Prozac: The Unhealthy Relationship between the Pharmaceutical Industry and Depression*. New York: New York University Press.

Helms, Robert, ed. 2002. *Guinea Pig Zero: An Anthology of the Journal for Human Research Subjects*. New Orleans: Garrett County.

Higby, George J., and Elaine C. Stroud, eds. 1990. *Pill Peddlers: Essays on the History of the Pharmaceutical Industry*. Madison: American Institute for the History of Pharmacy.

Hogshire, Jim. 1992. *Sell Yourself to Science*. Port Townsend, Wash.: Loompanics.

Hornblum, Allen M. 1998. *Acres of Skin: Human Experimentation at Holmesburg Prison*. New York: Routledge.

Jones, J. 1981. *Bad Blood: The Tuskegee Syphilis Experiment*. New York: Free Press.

Katz, Jay. 1972. *Experimentation with Human Beings*. New York: Russell Sage Foundation.

——. 1984. *The Silent World of Doctor and Patient*. New York: Free Press.

Kaufert, Joseph M., and John D. O'Neil. 1997. "Biomedical Rituals and Informed Consent: Native Canadians and the Negotiation of Clinical Trust." *Social Science Perspectives on Medical Ethics*, ed. George Weisz. Philadelphia: University of Pennsylvania Press.

Kleinman, Arthur. 1988. *The Illness Narratives: Suffering, Healing and the Human Condition*. New York: Basic.

Kleinman, Arthur, Veena Das, and Margaret Lock, eds. 2001. *Social Suffering*. Berkeley: University of California Press.

Kopytoff, L. 1985. "The Cultural Biography of Things: Commoditization as Process." *The Social Life of Things: Commodities in Cultural Perspective*, ed. Arjun Appadurai, 64–94. Cambridge: Cambridge University Press.

Lakoff, Andrew. 2005. *Pharmaceutical Reason: Medication and Psychiatric Knowledge in Argentina*. Cambridge: Cambridge University Press.

Lash, S., B. Szerszynski, and B. Wynne. 1996. *Risk, Environment and Modernity: Towards a New Ecology*. London: Sage.

Latour, Bruno. 1986. *Laboratory Life: The Construction of Scientific Facts*. Princeton: Princeton University Press.

——. 2004. *Politics of Nature: How to Bring the Sciences into Democracy*. Cambridge: Harvard University Press.

Lereder, Susan. 1992. "Orphans as Guinea Pigs: American Children and Medical Experimenters, 1890–1930." *In the Name of the Child: Health and Welfare, 1880–1940*, ed. Roger Cooter. London: Routledge.

——. 1995. *Subjected to Science: Human Experimentation in America before the Second World War*. Baltimore: Johns Hopkins University Press.

Levin, Betty. 1985. "Consensus and Controversy in the Treatment of Catastrophically Ill Newborn." *Which Babies Shall Live?*, ed. T. H. Murray and A. L. Caplan. Clifton, N.J.: Humana.

——. 1991. "Treatment Choice for Infants in the Neonatal Intensive Care Unit at Risk for AIDS." *Journal of the American Medical Association* 265, no. 22, 2976–81.

Levine, Robert J. 1998. *Ethics and Regulation of Clinical Research*, 2nd edn. Baltimore: Urban and Schwarzenberg.

Liebenau, Jonathan. 1987. *Medical Science and Medical Industry: The Formation of the American Pharmaceutical Industry*. Baltimore: Johns Hopkins University Press.

Lindenbaum, Shirley. 1979. *Kuru Sorcery: Disease and Danger in the New Guinea Highlands*. Palo Alto, Calif.: Mayfield.

Lindenbaum, Shirley, and Margaret Lock, eds. 1996. *Knowledge, Power and Practice: The Anthropology of Medicine and Everyday Life*. Berkeley: University of California Press.

Lock, Margaret. 1992. "Cultivating the Body: Anthropology and Epistemologies of Bodily Practice and Knowledge." *Annual Review of Anthropology* 22, 133–55.

Lock, Margaret, and Judith Farquhar, eds. 2007. *Beyond the Body Proper: Reading the Anthropology of Material Life*. Durham: Duke University Press.

Lock, Margaret, and Nancy Scheper-Hughes. 1987. "The Mindful Body: A Prolegomenon to Future Work in Medical Anthropology." *Medical Anthropology Quarterly* 1, no. 1, 6–41.

Lock, Margaret, Allan Young, and A. Cambrosio, eds. 1999. *Living and Working with the New Medical Technologies*. Cambridge: Cambridge University Press.

Lupton, Deborah. 1993. "Risk as a Moral Danger: The Social and Political Functions of Risk Discourse in Public Health." *International Journal of Health Services* 23, 425–35.

——. 1999. *Risk*. London: Routledge.

——, ed. 2000. *Risk and Sociocultural Theory: New Directions and Perspectives*. Cambridge: Cambridge University Press.

Macpherson, Crawford B. 1962. *The Political Theory of Possessive Individualism: Hobbes to Locke*. Oxford: Clarendon.

Mahoney, Tom. 1959. *The Merchants of Life: An Account of the American Pharmaceutical Industry*. New York: Harper and Brothers.

Markowitz, Gerald, and David Rosner. 2003. *Deceit and Denial: The Deadly Politics of Industrial Production*. Berkeley: University of California Press.

Marks, Harry. 1997. *The Progress of Experiment: Science and Therapeutic Reform in the United States, 1900–1990*. Cambridge: Cambridge University Press.

Marshall, Patricia. 1992. "Anthropology and Bioethics." *Medical Anthropology Quarterly* 6, no. 1, 49–73.

Marshall, Patricia, and Barbara Koenig. 2004. "Accounting for Culture in a Globalized Ethics." *Journal of Law, Medicine, and Ethics* 32, no. 2, 252–66.

Martin, Emily. 1994. *Flexible Bodies: Tracking Immunity in American Culture from the Days of Polio to the Age of AIDS*. Boston: Beacon.

Marx, Karl. 1976 [1867]. *Capital: A Critique of Political Economy*. London: Penguin.

Maskovsky, Jeff. 2000. " 'Fighting for Life': Poverty, AIDS, and Community Activism in Neo-liberal Philadelphia." Diss., Temple University.

Maskovsky, Jeff, and Judith Goode, eds. 2001. *New Poverty Studies: The Ethnography of Power, Politics, and Impoverished People in the United States*. New York: New York University Press.

McNeil, Paul M. 1992. *The Ethics and Politics of Human Experimentation*. Cambridge: Cambridge University Press.

Meyer, Peter B. 1974. *Drug Experiments on Prisoners*. Lexington, Mass: Lexington Books.

Mills, C. Wright. 1959. *The Power Elite*. New York: Oxford University Press.

Mintz, Sidney W. 1985. *Sweetness and Power: The Place of Sugar in Modern History*. New York: Viking.

Mitchell, Don. 2003. *Right to the City: Social Justice and the Fight for Public Space*. New York: Guilford.

Moerman, Daniel. 2000. "Cultural Variations in the Placebo Effect: Ulcers, Anxiety and Blood Pressure." *Medical Anthropology Quarterly* 14, 51–72.

Moore, Lisa Jean, and Matthew Schmidt. 1999. "On the Construction of Male Differences: Marketing Variations in Technosemen." *Men and Masculinities* 1, no. 4, 339–59.

Moreno, Jonathan. 2000. *Undue Risk: Secret State Experiments on Humans*. New York: W. H. Freeman.

Nash, June. 1986. *From Tank Town to High Tech: The Clash of Community and Industrial Cycles*. Albany: State University of New York Press.

Nugent, David. 2002. *Locating Capitalism in Time and Space: Global Restructuring, Politics, and Identity*. Stanford: Stanford University Press.

Oldani, Michael. 2004. "Thick Prescriptions: Towards an Interpretation of Pharmaceutical Sales Practices." *Medical Anthropology Quarterly* 18, 328–56.

Pappas, George. 1989. *The Magic City*. Ithaca: Cornell University Press.

Pappworth, M. H. 1967. *Human Guinea Pigs*. Boston: Beacon.

Parascandola, John. 1985. "Industrial Research Comes of Age." *Pharmacy in History* 27 (fall), 12–21.

———. 1998. *The Development of American Pharmacology: John Abel and the Shaping of a Discipline*. Baltimore: Johns Hopkins University Press.

Parker, Richard, and P. Aggleton, eds. 1999. *Culture, Society, and Sexuality: A Reader.* London: UCL Press.

Parker, Richard., R. M. Barbosa, and P. Aggleton, eds. 2000. *Framing the Sexual Subject: The Politics of Gender, Sexuality and Power.* Berkeley: University of California Press.

Patriquin, Martin. 2009. "Inside the Human Guinea Pig Capital of North America." *Macleans*, 25 August.

Petryna, Adriana. 2002. *Life Exposed: Biological Citizens after Chernobyl.* Princeton: Princeton University Press.

———. 2005. "Ethical Variability: Drug Development and Globalizing Clinical Trials." *American Ethnologist* 32, no. 2 (May), 183–97.

———. 2006. "Globalizing Human Subjects Research." *Global Pharmaceutics: Ethics, Markets and Practices*, ed. Adriana Petryna et al., 33–60. Durham: Duke University Press.

———. 2009. *When Experiments Travel: Clinical Trials and the Global Search for Human Subjects.* Princeton: Princeton University Press.

Polanyi, Karl. 1974. *The Great Transformation.* New York: Octagon.

Proctor, Robert N. 1985. *Racial Hygiene: Medicine under the Nazis.* Cambridge: Harvard University Press.

Rajan, Kaushink S. 2005. "Subjects of Speculation: Emergent Life Sciences and Market Logics in the United States and India." *American Anthropologist* 107, no. 1, 19–30.

———. 2006. *Biocapital: The Constitution of Postgenomic Life.* Durham: Duke University Press.

Rapp, Rayna. 1999. *Testing the Women, Testing the Fetus: The Social Impact of Amniocentesis in America.* New York: Routledge.

Reverby, Susan, ed. 2000. *Tuskegee Truths: Rethinking the Tuskegee Syphilis Study.* Chapel Hill: University of North Carolina Press.

Rhodes, Lorna A. 1991. *Emptying Beds: The Work of an Emergency Psychiatric Unit.* Berkeley: University of California Press.

Robotham, Don. 2005. *Culture, Society and Economy: Bringing Production Back In.* Thousand Oaks, Calif.: Sage.

Rose, Nikolas. 1996. "Governing 'Advanced' Liberal Democracies." *Foucault and Political Reason: Liberalism, Neo-liberalism, and Rationalities of Government*, ed. Andrew Barry, Thomas Osborne, and Nikolas Rose. Chicago: University of Chicago Press.

———. 2006. *The Politics of Life Itself: Biomedicine, Power, and Subjectivity in the Twenty-First Century.* Princeton: Princeton University Press.

Rosner, David, and Gerald Markowitz. 1991. *Deadly Dust: Silicosis and the Politics of Occupational Disease in Twentieth-Century America.* Princeton: Princeton University Press.

Rothman, David. 2000. *Strangers at the Bedside: A History of How Law and Bioethics Transformed Medical Decision Making.* New York: Basic.

Rutheiser, C. 1999. "Making Place in the Nonplace Urban Realm: Notes on the Revitalization of Downtown Atlanta." *Theorizing the City: The New Urban Anthropology Reader*, ed. S. Low. New Brunswick: Rutgers University Press.

Sassen, Saskia. 1992. "The Informal Economy." *Dual City: Restructuring New York*, ed. Manuel Castells and John Mollenkopf. New York: Russell Sage Foundation.

Scheper-Hughes, Nancy. 1996. "Body Trades: The Global Commerce for Transplant Surgery." *Current Anthropology* 41, February.

Scheper-Hughes, Nancy, and Loïc Wacquant, eds. 2002. *Commodifying Bodies*. Newbury Park, Calif.: Sage.

Sharff, Jagna. 1998. *King Kong on Fourth Street: Families and the Violence of Poverty in Lower East Side*. Boulder: Westview.

Sharp, Leslie. 2000. "The Commodification of the Body and Its Parts." *Annual Review of Anthropology* 29, 287–328

———. 2006. *Strange Harvest: Organ Transplants, Denatured Bodies, and the Transformed Self*. Berkeley: University of California Press.

———. 2007. *Bodies, Commodities and Biotechnologies: Death, Mourning, and Scientific Desire in the Realm of Human Organ Transfer*. New York: Columbia University Press.

Silverman, Milton, and Philip R. Lee. 1974. *Pills, Profits, and Politics*. Berkeley: University of California Press.

Singer, Merrill. 1994. "AIDS and the Health Crisis of the U.S. Urban Poor: The Perspective of Critical Medical Anthropology." *Social Science and Medicine* 39, no. 7, 931–48.

———. 1998. *The Political Economy of AIDS*. Amityville, N.Y.: Baywood.

———. 2006. *The Face of Social Suffering: Life History of a Street Drug Addict*. Prospect Heights, Ill.: Waveland.

Singer, Merrill, and Hans Baer, eds. 2009. *Killer Commodities: A Critical Anthropological Examination of Corporate Products and Public Health*. New York: Rowman and Littlefield.

Smith, Neil. 1996. *New Urban Frontier: Gentrification and the Revanchist City*. London: Routledge.

Starr, Paul. 1982. *The Social Transformations of American Medicine*. New York: Basic.

Stull, William J., and J. Fanning Madden. 1984. *Post-industrial Philadelphia: Structural Changes in the Metropolitan Economy*. Philadelphia: University of Pennsylvania Press.

Susser, Ida. 1982. *Norman Street: Poverty and Politics in an Urban Neighborhood*. New York: Oxford University Press.

———. 1988. "Directions in Research in Health and Industry." *Medical Anthropology Quarterly* 2, no. 3, 195–98.

———. 1996. "The Construction of Poverty and Homelessness in US Cities." *Annual Review of Anthropology* 25, 411–35.

Swann, John. 1984. *Academic Scientists and the Pharmaceutical Industry: Cooperative Research in Twentieth-Century America*. Baltimore: John Hopkins University Press.

———. 1995. "The Evolution of the American Pharmaceutical Industry." *Pharmacy in History* 37, no. 2, 76–86.

Temin, Peter. 1980. *Taking Your Medicine: Drug Regulation in the United States*. Cambridge: Harvard University Press.

Thompson, Edward Palmer. 1966. *The Making of the English Working Class*. New York: Vintage.

Treicheler, P. 2000. *How to Have Theory in an Epidemic: Cultural Chronicles of* AIDS. Durham: Duke University Press.

Turner, Victor. 1968. *The Drums of Affliction*. New York: Oxford University Press.

Vuckovic, Nancy, and Mark Nichter. 1997. "Changing Patterns of Pharmaceutical Practice in the United States." *Social Science Medicine* 44, 1285–1302.

Weinstein, Matthew. 2001. "A Public Culture for Guinea Pigs: US Human Research Subjects after the Tuskegee Study." *Sciences as Culture* 10 (June), 195–233.

Whyte, Susan Reynolds, Sjaak vand der Geest, and Anita Hardon. 1996. "The Anthropology of Pharmaceuticals: A Biographical Approach." *Annual Review of Anthropology* 25, 153–78.

——. 2002. *Social Lives of Medicines*. Cambridge: Cambridge University Press.

Wolf, Eric, and Sydel Silverman. 2001. *Building an Anthropology of the Modern World*. Berkeley: University of California Press.

Young, Allan. 1998. *The Harmony of Illusions: Invention of Post-traumatic Stress Disorder*. Princeton: Princeton University Press.

INDEX

Community Programs for Clinical Research on AIDS (CPCRA), 86, 87, 93

Corrigan, Oonagh, 73

Contract research organizations (CROs): conditions at, 15–22, 52; shift from industry trials to, 22; subjects recruited by, 23, 156

Data Safety Monitoring Board (DSMB), 89, 90

Di Leonardo, Michaela, 17

Douglas, Mary, 69, 72

Drugs: adverse reactions to, 7, 65, 66, 73, 79, 89, 165, 170; anaphylactic reaction to, 141; animal testing of, 3, 65, 138; antiretroviral therapy, 88; approval process for, 21, 88; backbone, 148; bioequivalence tests, 5; blockbuster, 60; development of, 3, 97; dosing of, 28; efficacy of, 21, 27; expanded access to, 88, 110, 116; ethical, 132, 133; experimental, 75, 166; first in man, 5, 9, 16; genetic, 79; long-term effects of, 7, 82, 170; "me too," 16, 62, 166; pipeline, 2, 80; pricing of, 3; proprietary, 132, 133; protease inhibitor, 88, 109, 110; Prozac 76; psychotropic, 6, 76, 79; safety of, 27; synergistic interactions of, 82, 165. *See also* Clinical trials

Elliott, Carl, 155, 163, 168

Embodiment: disembodied self, 11; professional subject's scars, 10, 29, 41; theories of, 10

Ethnography of paid trial subjects, 3, 11, 70, 164, 167

Food and Drug Administration (FDA): clinical trials on prisoners and, 125; Harris Kaufert Act, 126; Pure Food and Drug Act (1906), 132; neoliberal regulatory environment and, 7–8, 166

Financial compensation: in cash, 16; for HIV clinical trials, 13, 91, 93–95; to increase enrollment, 2; for low-skill jobs, 161; market recruitment and, 41, 122, 135, 157; pro-rated, 81, 155; risk perception and, 6, 30; subjects' addiction to, 5, 36; taxes paid on, 46

Gelsinger, Jesse, 155, 165

Guinea Pig Zero, 12, 49–51; professional guinea pigs culture and, 39, 52; sense of humor of, 73

Giddens, Anthony, 67

Glaxo Smith Kline (GSK), 11, 42, 77, 168

Helms, Robert, 11, 38, 49, 53, 74, 167–69

Hippocratic Oath, 123

HIV clinical trials, 98–99, 101, 113–15, 158; African Americans in, 3, 90, 143; community empowerment and, 103, 105–10; financial compensation to volunteers in, 13, 91, 93–95; informed consent for, 153; Latinos in, 3, 90; medical trust and, 143; minority enrollment in, 3, 85, 90, 94, 97, 143; motivations to participate in, 5, 91, 93–95, 119; patients' quality of life and, 118; politics of drug development and, 85, 147; risk perception and, 100, 102–4, 144–45, 153; SMART trial, 86, 87, 88, 93, 144; survivor narrative and, 98; Wistar trial, 87, 116. *See also* CBTO

Hogshire, Jim, 5

Holmesburg Prison, 10

Hornblum, Allen, 10

Human experimentation: abuses of, 69, 123; ethics of, 122, 124, 125; as exploitation, 7, 61, 62, 140, 154, 165; Helsinki Declaration, 7, 154; under Nazis, 124, 156; Nuremberg Code and, 149; in orphanages, 122; of poor and vulnerable, 121, 123, 154, 156; on prisoners, 7, 66, 122, 125, 154; in Second

World War, 124, 156; at Tuskegee, 12, 123, 124, 143. *See also* Belmont Report; HIV clinical trials; IRBs; Professional guinea pigs

Industrial Workers of the World, 53, 167
Informed consent: changes to, 139; confusing language of, 139, 156; inability to give proper, 125; as legal document, 151; regulation of, 125; in Phase I trials, 28, 74; process for, 1, 28, 73, 137, 139, 156; subjects' understanding of, 137–43; uncoerced, 4, 139, 156
IRBs (institutional review boards), 2, 155, 165; of CBTO, 89, 145, 148–50; for hire, 22

Jefferson Hospital, 12, 28, 53, 58, 62, 137, 168
Jones, James, 12
Johns Hopkins University, 1

Koenig, Barbara, 19

Lereder, Susan, 122
Libenau, Jonathan, 130–35
Lupton, Deborah, 67

Marks, John, 123, 126
Marshall, Patricia, 19
Martin, Emily, 160
Merck, 131, 168

National Commission for the Protection of Human Subjects of Biomedical and Behavioral Research, 7, 124, 154
National Institutes of Health (NIH), 87, 94, 147
National Research Act, 124

Oldani, Michael, 18
Organ transplantation, 8

Paid volunteers, 9, 10, 45
Petryna, Adriana, 18, 71, 122
Phase I clinical trials, 21; age limit for, 11, 56; alternates in, 32; gender bias in, 23; in India, 136; as mild torture economy, 2, 46; penalties for quitting, 55; in Philadelphia, 33, 59, 60; recruitment for, 41, 66, 122, 125; report cards on, 52, 77; schedule of, 32, 57; social organization of, 56, 59, 122, 126. *See also* Financial compensation; Healthy paid subjects; HIV clinical trials; Recruitment
Phase II and III clinical trials, 3, 13, 21, 88
Pharmaceutical industry: academia and, 1, 22, 131, 135; centralization of, 134; globalization of, 121, 163; history of, 130–35; liability and, 76, 142, 164; marketing by, 7, 150; profits of, 7; regulation of, 134
Philadelphia: biomedical research in, 122; clinical trials in, 33, 59, 60; deindustrialization of, 128–29; pharmaceutical industry in, 11, 122, 129–31; service economy of, 122, 135
Professional guinea pigs, 10, 47, 49, 69, 82, 122; African American, 12, 54, 163, 170; altruism of, 2, 30; anarchists as, 11, 12, 26, 39, 61, 77; backgrounds of, 12, 29–32; boredom of, 2, 16; careers of, 25, 79; collective action by, 56–60, 141; community of, 11, 26, 34–36; compliance by, 2, 6, 25, 155; death of, 1; dehumanization of, 6, 140; diversity among, 13, 162; geographical mobility of, 42; ideology of, 36, 61–63; income of, 5, 31; invisibility of, 12, 17; Latino, 12, 29, 40; motivations of, 5, 30; pain experienced by, 16, 162; pharmaceutical industry distrust of, 142; professionalization of, 3, 5, 7, 13, 16, 24–26, 126, 157; recommendations for safeguarding, 165–66;

Professional guinea pigs (*cont.*)
resistance by, 6, 11, 53–63; rights of,
2, 165; sex workers likened to, 11, 48;
shared interests of, 157; social identity
of, 2, 12, 31, 45, 46, 50, 48, 5; socialization among, 73, 79; solidarity of, 11;
strikes by, 12, 53, 41, 61; survey of, 12,
15, 29–30; women as, 13, 61–63;
workplace organizing by, 58–60
Public Health Service, 123

Randomized clinical trials (RCTs), 22, 27;
experimental design and, 21, 65, 122,
125; placebo, 27; randomization in,
27, 153; standard, 128; validity of,
126–27
Recruitment, 25–28, 126; for Phase I
clinical trials, 41, 66, 122, 125; reliance on professional trial subjects
and, 24, 54, 161; screening and, 22
Reverby, Susan, 12
Risk, 2, 6, 75–77; beliefs about body
cleansing practices and, 80–82; of
dangerous trades, 48; denial of, 65,
66; effects of continuous trial par-

ticipation on, 78; financial compensation and, 7, 66, 69, 71, 78, 80; long-
term, 8, 48, 66, 74, 78, 79; risk exposure despite, 7, 82; shaping by local
knowledge of, 73, 80–82; short-term,
74; theories of, 67–72
Robert Wood Johnson Foundation, 86
Roche, Ellen, 1, 155, 165
Rose, Nikolas, 18

Salvarsan, 131
Scheper-Huges, Nancy, 8
Sharp, Leslie, 8
Singer, Merrill, 69, 71
Sleep deprivation studies, 6, 79
Susser, Ida, 69, 94

Temple University 11
Tipranavir, 116, 147, 148

University of Pennsylvania, 86, 87, 90
Upjohn, 127, 131

Wyeth, 11, 130, 168

Roberto Abadie is a visiting scholar with the Health
Sciences Doctoral Programs at the Graduate Center,
City University of New York.

Library of Congress Cataloging-in-Publication Data
Abadie, Roberto.
The professional guinea pig : Big Pharma and the
risky world of human subjects / Roberto Abadie.
p. cm.
Includes bibliographical references and index.
ISBN 978-0-8223-4814-6 (cloth : alk. paper)
ISBN 978-0-8223-4823-8 (pbk. : alk. paper)
1. Drugs—Testing. 2. Drugs—United States—
Testing. 3. Human experimentation in medicine—
United States. I. Title.
RM301.27.A22 2010
615'.19—dc22   2010004457